ZONE
PERFECT
MEALS
IN MINUTES

Other books by Barry Sears, Ph.D.

The Zone
Mastering the Zone

ZONE PERFECT MEALS IN MINUTES

150 Fast and Simple Healthy Recipes from the Bestselling Author of THE ZONE and MASTERING THE ZONE

BARRY SEARS, Ph.D.

ReganBooks
An Imprint of HarperCollinsPublishers

HarperCollins books may be purchased for educational, business, or sales promotional use. For information please write: Special Markets Department, HarperCollins Publishers, Inc., 10 East 53rd Street, New York, NY 10022.

FIRST EDITION

Designed by Nancy Singer Olaguera

Library of Congress Cataloging-in-Publication Data
Sears, Barry, 1947–
    Zone-perfect meals in minutes / by Barry Sears.
      p. cm.
    Includes index.
    ISBN 0-06-039241-X
    1. Reducing diets—Recipes. I.Title.
  RM222.2.S393   1997
  613.2'5—dc21   97-31133

97 98 99 00 01 ❖/RRD 10 9 8 7 6 5 4 3 2 1

CONTENTS

Appendixes:

ACKNOWLEDGMENTS

Rarely is any work done alone, and this book is no exception. As usual, primary thanks must be given to my wife, Lynn Sears, and my brother, Doug Sears, not only for their editorial comments, but also for their valuable feedback on how to better communicate Zone concepts to the general public.

Other important contributions have resulted from the thousands of responses from readers of the Zone books. Also, many thanks must go to Todd Silverstein for his exceptionally insightful editing of the manuscript and his constant support.

Much of the early part of this book is inspired by the educational materials developed for teaching Type II diabetics how to use the Zone Diet as part of their treatment programs. But all this would be for naught without the recipes skillfully created and tested by Scott C. Lane, who also crafted the recipes for *Mastering the Zone*. Scott combines the rare talent of being a gourmet chef with a background in food technology. His contributions have been invaluable. The results of his work are recipes that are not only great-tasting, but have powerful hormonal benefits that can be considered the cutting edge of food technology for the twenty-first century.

I also want to thank my friends Dr. Michael Eades and Dr. Michael Norder for their unique insights into the role of diet and hormonal response. Furthermore, much credit must also go to the medical staff at Eicotech consisting of Dr. Paul Kahl and Dr. Eric Freeland for their extremely valuable contributions.

Finally, and most important, my deepest thanks must be given to Judith Regan, who had the courage to publish the first of the Zone books, and who has given invaluable insight into how to best communicate these concepts to the general public. Without her continuing support, the concept of the Zone might never have come to light.

WOULD YOU BUY
THIS DRUG?

What if you could buy a drug that keeps you mentally focused throughout the day? What if the same drug could increase your physical stamina, leaving you with excess energy when you get home? What if it would eliminate hunger between meals? What if it could reduce the likelihood of developing chronic diseases that rob life of its dignity? Would you buy such a drug? Of course.

Would you be startled to learn that such a drug already exists? That the side effects of taking this drug are the loss of excess body fat at the maximum rate possible, and a slowing of the aging process? Best of all, this wonder drug won't cost you a thing. Why? Because you are already taking it every day.

This magical elixir I am describing is food. The food you eat is probably the most powerful drug you will ever encounter. But to use this drug correctly you have to apply the hormonal rules about food that haven't changed in the past 40 million years, and are unlikely to change any time soon. Beware, the door swings both ways on the application of these hormonal rules. Used correctly, food becomes the exceptionally powerful drug that mankind has searched millenniums for. Used incorrectly, on the other hand, food can become your worst nightmare, as tens of millions of Americans have already discovered.

How does this drug work? Simply stated, you must learn how to administer food in the appropriate combination, at the right time, and in the correct dosage to keep the hormone insulin in a tight zone—not too high, not too low. That's the definition of the Zone. The Zone is about maintaining a steady range of insulin in your bloodstream, and food is the only drug known to medical science that you can use to reach that goal. The Zone Diet is the prescription you need to use that drug (i.e., food) correctly.

In my first book, *The Zone,* I outlined the science behind my approach of using food as a drug to control insulin. My second book, *Mastering the Zone,* was a how-to book to apply the principles of the Zone to daily living. This third book addresses the greatest enemy to reaching the Zone—time. The biggest complaint about the Zone Diet is that it takes too much time. No longer. If you follow a few simple rules and use the recipes provided in this book, it will now take you only minutes to enter the Zone.

Why has the Zone Diet become the rage of Hollywood? Why is the Zone Diet followed by world-class athletes? Why is the Zone Diet used by millions of average Americans like yourself? Because it works. That's also why the Zone Diet has become the scourge of the nutritional establishment, which has told you for the past fifteen years that eating bagels and pasta is a surefire way to reach nutritional nirvana. Yet, no one can say with a straight face that Americans are healthier now than they were fifteen years ago.

So if you are one of the millions of Americans who are not happy with what has happened to your body and your health in the past fifteen years, this book will be your primer on using a powerful drug, food, to get into the Zone, quickly and effortlessly. Consider this book a lifelong prescription for a better quality of life.

You can, if you wish, jump directly to the recipes in Chapter 6 to start your Zone prescription. But if you want a little more background on the Zone, then read the next few short chapters.

HORMONAL THINKING VERSUS CALORIC THINKING

This chapter will give you a capsule summary of the concepts that are the foundation of the Zone, as detailed in both *The Zone* (1995) and *Mastering the Zone* (1997).

I have come to realize that two things in life are visceral: our beliefs about nutrition and religion. Both generate passionate feelings, and neither responds well to challenge. Both have also been responsible for the deaths of more people than all the wars mankind has waged thus far. Diet and religion are fightin' words.

As part of our war on obesity, Americans have been told for the past fifteen years that fat is the enemy, and we have lined up as very willing soldiers to wage war against fat. If fat is the enemy, we should have won the war by now. Today we are eating less fat than at any other time in our history, yet we have become the fattest people on the face of the earth.

This is why health authorities like Dr. C. Everett Koop have called obesity the greatest public health crisis currently facing the nation. Why? As readers of *The Zone* already know, this epidemic explosion in obesity may be just the tip of the iceberg, a precursor to an unprecedented increase in chronic disease in the next decade.

What went wrong with our noble war against fat? Doesn't fat cause you to become fat? No. Unfortunately it never has, and it never will. The real cause of increased accumulation of body fat (and our inability to shed it) is the excess production of the hormone insulin. This same excess of insulin also accelerates the likelihood of heart disease, diabetes, and possibly cancer.

We're losing the war against obesity because nutritionists continue to think calorically, instead of looking at food from a hormonal perspective.

You can sum up caloric thinking in a single phrase: "If no fat touches my lips, then no fat will reach my hips." Seductive thinking, but alas, it's not true. Hormonal thinking, on the other hand, says: "It's excess insulin that makes you fat and keeps you fat." Since fat has no effect on insulin, our perceived enemy, fat, is really a neutral bystander in the war on obesity. And this is one war that we are rapidly losing on every front.

Hormonal thinking, which is the foundation of the Zone Diet, can be summarized by the following points. Each of these points may challenge the very core of what you think you know about nutrition.

1. **It is impossible for dietary fat alone to make you fat.** It is the hormone insulin that makes you fat and keeps you fat. How do you increase insulin levels? By eating too many fat-free carbohydrates or too many calories at any one meal. Americans have done both in the past fifteen years. People tend to forget that the best way to fatten cattle and pigs is to raise their insulin levels by feeding them lots and lots of low-fat grain. The best way to fatten humans is to raise their insulin levels by feeding them lots and lots of low-fat grain, but now in the form of pasta and bagels.

2. **Your stomach is politically incorrect.** The stomach is basically a vat of acid that breaks all food into its basic components. From that perspective, one Snickers bar has the same amount of carbohydrate as two ounces of pasta. Most people would not eat four Snickers bars at one sitting, but they would have no problem eat-

ing eight ounces of pasta. Your stomach can't tell the difference. And the more carbohydrates you eat, the more insulin you produce. And the more insulin you produce, the fatter you become.

3. **Not everyone is genetically the same**. About 25 percent of the U.S. population is genetically lucky because they have a low insulin response to carbohydrates. These people will never become fat, and they will always do well on any high-carbohydrate diet whether it's pasta, Snickers, or Twinkies. Unfortunately, the other 75 percent of the U.S. population isn't so lucky. As they increase the amount of fat-free carbohydrates in their diet, they increase the production of insulin.

   Next time you look at that breakfast bagel, ask the question: "Do I feel lucky?" You have a 25 percent chance that you might be. On the other hand, you have a 75 percent chance that your morning bagel will be your worst hormonal nightmare.

4. **Ten thousand years ago there were no grains on the face of the earth.** During mankind's evolution, our ancestors were exposed to two food groups only: low-fat protein and low-density carbohydrates (fruits and vegetables). As a result, this is what we are genetically designed to eat. When grains were first introduced into the human diet 10,000 years ago, the archaeological record clearly reflects three immediate and dramatic changes in grain-eating societies:
   a. Mankind shrank in height from lack of adequate protein.
   b. Diseases of "modern civilization," such as heart attacks, first appeared.
   c. Obesity first became apparent.

   Nowhere is this clearer than in the comparison of Egyptian mummies to the skeletons of Neo-Paleolithic man. Ancient Egyptians were shorter by about six inches than Neo-Paleolithic man, probably because the Egyptians' protein consumption had dropped so dramatically.

More ominously for us, ancient Egyptian medical textbooks dating back as far as 3,500 years ago describe heart disease in frightening detail. Their medical descriptions of heart disease are confirmed when one examines those mummies with preserved visceral tissue that show extensive atherosclerotic lesions, even through the average Egyptian lifespan was only twenty years.

Finally, it is estimated that the extent of obesity in ancient Egypt was similar to the extent of obesity currently found in the United States. We can determine this from the excess amount of skin folds found around the midsections of preserved Egyptian mummies. (Keep in mind that the diet eaten by the ancient Egyptians was very similar to the diet now recommended by the U.S. government for every American. Talk about history repeating itself.)

5. **It takes fat to burn fat.** This statement makes no sense if you are thinking calorically, but it makes perfect sense if you are thinking hormonally. Fat acts like a control rod in a nuclear reactor, slowing down the entry rate of carbohydrates into the bloodstream, and thereby decreasing the production of insulin. Fat also sends a hormonal signal to the brain, telling you to stop eating, which is another way it reduces insulin production.

    Since it's excess insulin that makes you fat, having more fat in the diet becomes an important tool for reducing insulin. The best type of fat to add to your meals? Monounsaturated fat, like olive oil, guacamole, almonds, and macadamia nuts.

6. **You can use food as a hormonal ATM card.** The average American male or female carries a minimum of 100,000 calories of stored body fat on their bodies at any one time. To put this in perspective, this amount of stored body fat is equivalent to eating 1,700 pancakes for breakfast. That's a pretty big breakfast. In fact, the calories you need for your daily energy are already stored in your body. What you need is a hormonal ATM card to release this stored fat for energy. The Zone Diet is that hormonal ATM card,

allowing you to access this massive amount of energy already stored in your body.

7. **The number-one predictor of heart disease is not high cholesterol, not high blood pressure, but elevated levels of insulin.** How can you tell if you have elevated levels of insulin? Look in the mirror. If you're fat and shaped like an apple, you have elevated insulin levels, and you are probably fast-tracking to an early heart attack. But you can still be thin and have elevated insulin. How can you tell? You have high triglycerides and low HDL cholesterol. This is why high-carbohydrate, low-fat diets can be extremely dangerous to cardiovascular patients even if they lose weight, because they often also see an increase in triglycerides and a decrease in HDL cholesterol levels.

8. **Carbohydrates are a drug.** Make no mistake about it. Your body needs some carbohydrate at every meal for optimal brain function. But like any drug, too much will give rise to toxic side effects. The toxic side effect of consuming too much carbohydrate at any meal is an overproduction of insulin, and that can be very dangerous to your health.

The central theme of the Zone Diet is to understand the importance of thinking of food hormonally, rather than calorically. Once you do so, you begin to understand why virtually every dietary recommendation of the U.S. government and leading nutritionists is hormonally wrong (and maybe dead wrong) for millions of Americans.

All that remains for you is to get into the Zone as easily and as quickly as possible. That's what this book is all about. But before we begin getting into the Zone, a little background on nutrition is needed to explain how and why the Zone Diet works.

===================== (3) =====================

WHAT IS FOOD?

Food can be divided into three groups: protein, carbohydrate, and fat. What these food groups are and how they affect the Zone Diet are the keys to understanding what and how you must eat to get and stay in the Zone.

PROTEIN

Protein comes primarily from animal sources because animals are very efficient concentrators of protein compared to plants. Protein levels in plants, on the other hand, are usually very low and, unfortunately, often require you to eat massive and unrealistic amounts of vegetable sources to obtain adequate protein intake (while also consuming massive amounts of carbohydrates that take you out of the Zone). Eating adequate protein is essential to health, because eating less than adequate protein is equivalent to protein malnutrition. But while virtually no one in America suffers from caloric malnutrition, a surprising number of people today suffer from protein malnutrition because they have eliminated protein from the diet and replaced it with increasing amounts of grains and pasta in their relentless effort to reduce dietary fat.

Why do you have to have adequate protein? Your body's immune system, the integrity of all your tissues, each of the body's cells, the enzymes (the engines of life) contained in each cell, and the amount of your muscle mass all depend on having adequate levels of new incoming protein, since you are losing protein every day through normal metabolism. If you don't have at least an equal amount of protein coming into the body to balance the amount that is being constantly lost from the body, you have protein malnutrition. Protein malnutrition can be insidious, leading to a decrease in the ability of your immune system to fight infection. You will also lose muscle mass as your body cannibalizes existing muscle in a losing effort to keep up with the demand for new protein building blocks for your immune system and new enzyme formation.

The key to the Zone Diet is to ensure that adequate amounts of protein are being supplied to your body like an intravenous drug that is delivered throughout the day in relatively controlled amounts based on your own unique protein requirements.

Notice, too, that you need *adequate*, not excessive protein. The Zone Diet is *not* a high-protein diet, but rather a protein-adequate diet. In fact, the Zone Diet has absolutely no relationship to the high-protein diets of the 1970s (this is explained in far greater detail in Chapter 13). Simply stated, no one should ever eat more protein than his or her body requires, but no one should ever eat less.

To make the picture a little more complex, not all protein is the same. On the Zone Diet, you want to keep the amount of saturated fat to a minimum. Therefore your primary source of protein will consist of low-fat choices such as chicken, fish, turkey, egg whites, low-fat cottage cheese, tofu, soybean imitation meat products, and isolated protein powders as opposed to bacon, steaks, and sausages.

Besides meeting the needs I have described above, protein also plays another critical hormonal role—it stimulates the release of the hormone called glucagon. Glucagon is a mobilization hormone that allows your body to use stored energy, both fat and carbohydrate, as energy sources.

CARBOHYDRATES

Carbohydrates come from plants and trees. Examples are grains (the basis of all pastas, breads, and cereals), or vegetables, or fruits.

In human nutrition, there is no such thing as an essential carbohydrate! You don't need to eat carbohydrates to live. This was demonstrated in 1927 when a noted Arctic explorer, Vihajalmur Stefansson and a colleague, confined themselves in a hospital ward for a year, eating only protein and fat, and no carbohydrates whatsoever. After one year on this diet, they were both perfectly normal.

Although you can live without carbohydrate, this is not true for protein or fat, as the human body cannot make essential protein (i.e., essential amino acids) and essential fat (i.e., essential fatty acids), and therefore these must be obtained in the diet if you are to survive. On the other hand, the body can make carbohydrate (necessary for brain function) from both protein and fat.

A complex carbohydrate is simply a large quantity of simple sugars strung together and looks something like this:

—glucose—O—glucose—O—glucose—O—glucose—O—glucose—

This is the configuration of pasta, starches, bagels, or cereals at the molecular level. Notice that a typical complex carbohydrate is simply a simple sugar (glucose) held together by an oxygen bond. These oxygen bonds are broken down in the stomach, thus allowing a complex carbohydrate to be absorbed.

How quickly this breakdown occurs determines how fast your blood sugar level rises. This is very important because it's the combination of the amount of carbohydrates you eat and the speed with which they enter into the bloodstream that dictate how much of insulin is produced.

The average American currently consumes the carbohydrate equivalent of more than two cups of sugar per day. This is because all carbohydrates, no matter how complex they might be when they enter your mouth, must be broken down to simple sugars to be absorbed.

Your stomach is politically incorrect because it can't tell the difference between a bagel, pasta, or cotton candy. And the more carbohydrates you consume, the more insulin you make.

Insulin (unlike glucagon) is a storage hormone. One of its functions is to push incoming calories into cells. And any excess carbohydrates or protein that can't be stored immediately are converted to fat. Insulin will then drive this newly converted fat into your fat cells for storage.

The Zone Diet is based on keeping glucagon and insulin balanced at every meal. This means maintaining the appropriate balance of protein and carbohydrate at every meal.

FATS

Finally, what about fat? Fats come from both animal and plant sources. There are three types of fat: saturated fat, which is solid at room temperature; monounsaturated fat, which is liquid at room temperature but solid in the freezer; and polyunsaturated fat, which remains a liquid even when frozen. An example of saturated fat is butter, a monounsaturated fat is olive oil, and a polyunsaturated fat is soybean oil. Since all your cells are composed of fat, the ratio of these types of fat in your diet will determine how effectively your body's cell membranes function. There is a fluidity zone (not too viscous, but not too fluid) that allows membranes to operate at optimal efficiency. This is the reason why the Zone Diet recommends the use of primarily monounsaturated fat.

Hormonally, fat has no direct effect on insulin or glucagon, but it does affect their balance by slowing down the absorption rate of any carbohydrate into the bloodstream, thereby decreasing insulin production. Furthermore, fat plays a critical role, because it provides the building blocks (essential fatty acids) for the production of the most important hormones in your body, called eicosanoids.

As explained in greater detail in *The Zone,* there are both "good" and "bad" eicosanoids, and their balance will determine whether your body works at peak efficiency or suffers from disease. As with insulin and glucagon, it's a matter of balance. And what controls this balance? The ratio of insulin and glucagon in your bloodstream determines whether your body makes "good" or "bad" eicosanoids.

The Zone Diet keeps all three hormonal systems (insulin, glucagon, and eicosanoids) working smoothly by treating food with the same respect that you would treat a prescription drug.

Preparing meals based on hormonal thinking may seem like a radical new approach to eating. So radical, in fact, that you might think no one has ever done it before in human history. As you read the next chapter, you will be surprised to learn just who has been eating in the Zone for a long time.

4

WHO ACTUALLY EATS IN THE ZONE?

Balancing your protein and carbohydrate to maintain insulin in a tight zone might sound almost impossible at first. Yet your grandmother had no problem doing it. Remember what your grandmother told you (or should have told you) about food? Probably these four simple rules.

1. **Eat small meals throughout the day.** One of the best ways to maintain insulin levels in the Zone is not to eat too much carbohydrate or protein at any one meal. Although carbohydrate has a powerful effect on stimulating insulin, protein can also stimulate its release. By not eating too much of either at any one meal, you are well on your way to the Zone. One of the frightening consequences of having the cheapest food on the face of the earth is that Americans have come to expect massive portions of food at every meal. And in the last fifteen years they have gotten their wish, but with a correspondingly massive increase in insulin production.

2. **Have some protein at every meal**. Protein's primary hormonal role is to stimulate the release of glucagon, which is a mobilization hormone. Glucagon also does a real bang-up job on control-

15

ling insulin output. Therefore, if you really want to get to the Zone, protein is your passport. But be careful about eating too much protein and remember the palm-of-your-hand rule discussed in *Mastering the Zone:* At any one meal, never consume any more protein than can fit on the palm of your hand (and no thicker than the palm of your hand). Your body simply can't handle any more at a meal, and any excess protein at a meal is converted to fat.

3. **Always eat your fruits and vegetables.** Any one can eat one cup of pasta, but it's hard work to eat six cups of steamed broccoli. Yet both contain the same amount of carbohydrates (due to the large amounts of fiber and water they contain which dilute out the carbohydrate). Why? Because fruits and vegetables are low-density carbohydrates. By eating primarily low-density carbohydrates, such as fruits and vegetables, you set up a natural control system that helps control the total amount of carbohydrates being consumed at any one meal. In addition, the fiber (especially if it's soluble fiber) in low-density carbohydrates helps slow down the rate of entry of carbohydrates into the bloodstream, thus lowering insulin secretion. On the other hand, grains, starches, pasta, and bagels are very high-density carbohydrates (which means it's very easy to overconsume them). This is why I recommend using high-density carbohydrates in moderation, as condiments, if you want to control insulin.

   Remember when your grandmother told you that you couldn't leave the table until you finished all your vegetables? She was simply being a good Zone coach.

4. **Take your cod liver oil.** Nothing is more disgusting than cod liver oil. However, it contains a special fatty acid called eicosapentaenoic acid, or EPA, that does a very good job of keeping insulin under control by affecting eicosanoids. You can still take cod liver oil like your grandmother did, but a better choice today is eating salmon, which is rich in that same fatty acid, but tastes a lot better.

Now, look at your grandmother's four Zone rules and compare them to what nutrition "experts" are advocating today. According to the U.S. Department of Agriculture Food Pyramid you are supposed to get most of your calories from breads, grains, starches, and pasta. A typical recommended daily menu might include a bagel for breakfast, pasta for lunch, and probably more pasta for dinner. By eating bountiful amounts of these recommended "healthy" foods, you may find it very easy to have large meals (at least in carbohydrate content) throughout the day: the first violation of your grandmother's rules.

Remember that famous commercial in which Clara demanded to know, "Where's the beef?" We could paraphrase her now and ask, "Where's the protein?" Because protein contains fat, it almost never appears at most breakfasts, rarely appears at lunch, and finally may make an almost apologetic appearance at dinner. Another violation of your grandmother's rules to have some protein at *every* meal.

Why eat lots of fruits and vegetables? Where do you think you get your vitamins and minerals from? They are found primarily in fruits and vegetables, not breads, starches, and pasta. In the land of plenty, we suffer from a massive underconsumption of fruits and vegetables, and a gross overconsumption of pasta and bagels. No wonder vitamin sales are booming.

Finally, what about cod liver oil? Your grandmother didn't know how or why it worked. It just seemed to work. We now know the fatty acids in cod liver oil favorably change the levels of eicosanoids.

OK, so the Zone Diet was fine for your grandmother, but that was nearly two generations ago. Is there anyone who eats in the Zone today? Actually, the French do. No one has ever accused the French of not eating well, yet they don't have the rampant obesity we have in this country, and their rate of heart disease is half of what it is in America. This is why our nutritional "experts" hate the French. They smoke, they drink, they don't exercise, they eat lots of fat, and their worst sin is that they seem to have a good time when they eat.

In reality, the French are Zoners. They eat a balance of protein to carbohydrate at every meal. They eat primarily fruits and vegetables, they eat in moderation, and they are not afraid of fat, especially in the form of sauces. And therein lies one of the secrets of French cooking—the sauces. And their drinking? Well, every time they drink wine (which the body treats like a carbohydrate), they always have a protein chaser (like cheese). If you ate gourmet French meals three times a day with slight adaptations, I guarantee you would be in the Zone.

The bottom line is that (1) you are genetically designed to eat a Zone Diet, (2) your grandmother told you to eat a Zone Diet, and (3) the French have demonstrated that the Zone Diet is really the pinnacle of gourmet cooking.

Now that you have had a basic primer on nutrition, all that remains is to teach you some very simple Zone rules. Once you know these easy rules, you will be well on your way to reaching the Zone.

5

ZONE RULES

Any drug use comes with certain rules and instructions to follow. The Zone Diet is no different. Does this mean Zone rules hard to understand? Not at all. Just follow your grandmother's four simple dietary rules as I outlined in the previous chapter. To make it even easier for yourself, for the first two weeks you're on the Zone Diet, simply put starch, pasta, cereals, bread, and bagels out of sight. During these two weeks, you will get your carbohydrates the old-fashioned way, from fruits and vegetables.

Now each time you sit down for a meal simply divide your plate into three equal sections. In one section you will put a portion of low-fat protein (chicken, turkey, fish, etc.) that is no larger than the palm of your hand (and no thicker than the palm). Fill the other two-thirds of the plate with fruits and vegetables. Then add a dash of monounsaturated fat (olive oil, slivered almonds, guacamole, etc.).

You're probably telling yourself, "It can't be this easy." Well, it is. Just do it at every meal and snack and you'll be pretty close to the center of the Zone throughout the day.

What if you want even greater precision? Can you achieve it? Yes, it's called the Zone food block method and its use is explained in greater detail in *Mastering the Zone*. Since different foods have different densities of protein, carbohydrate, and fat, what the Zone food

19

block method does is put them on an equal footing by standardizing the amount of protein, carbohydrate, and fat in each block. If you don't want to bother to calculate your individual block requirements, keep in mind that the average American male requires four blocks of each (protein, carbohydrate, and fat) at every meal, whereas the average American female will require three blocks of each at every meal. (In fact, my latest clinical trials with Type II diabetics have led me to conclude that no adult should consume fewer than three blocks per meal.) No minicomputer required.

I have taken most of the foods you will ever eat and broken them down into Zone food blocks, and these are listed in Appendix B. Just remember to look up the amounts of your favorite foods that constitute one Zone food block, and as you reconstruct your Zone meal, just make the number of protein blocks equal the number of carbohydrate blocks, and then add an equal number of fat blocks.

If you are going to err in making a Zone-Perfect meal, then do so in the fat blocks, since fat has no effect on insulin. Furthermore, always pay close attention to the amount of carbohydrates you're adding to a meal, as you can use up your carbohydrate block allotment very quickly, especially if you are using high-density carbohydrates.

Another important Zone rule on meal timing. Never let more than five hours go by without eating a Zone meal or snack. Remember, the best time to eat is when you are not hungry.

Finally, there's exercise. Exercise will lower insulin levels, so it should be part of your Zone lifestyle. However, I like to apply the 80/20 rule to exercise. Most (more than 80 percent) of your insulin control will come from the diet, and a much smaller part (less than 20 percent) will come from exercise. The best exercise? Try walking 30 minutes every day. Just like the Zone Diet, exercise works only if you do it consistently.

To show you how easy and delicious Zone meals can be, the next chapter features 150 balanced Zone-Perfect meals, many of which can be prepared in minutes.

150 ZONE-PERFECT MEALS

This chapter is probably the reason you bought this book. These Zone-Perfect meals were designed by Scott C. Lane, an exceptionally talented culinary expert who is also trained in the most advanced food technology. Each meal not only looks great and tastes delicious, but it is also designed to control insulin levels for the next four to six hours. This is the definition of a Zone-Perfect meal. Each meal has been crafted with the same kind of precision that pharmaceuticals use in manufacturing their drugs.

Furthermore, these meals have been constructed so that you can reduce their cooking times by nearly 50 percent by substituting frozen vegetables in place of fresh vegetables. (Birds Eye frozen vegetables are a good commercial source since they often contain combinations of several Zone-favorable vegetables.) Each Zone-Perfect meal is designed to provide four blocks of protein, carbohydrate, and fat. This is the typical size for an American male, whereas the typical American female would require the slightly smaller meal using only three blocks.

As I explained in *Mastering the Zone*, Zone meals are incredibly flexible. Each recipe is organized into Zone food blocks, so that with a quick turn to the Appendix, you can modify any Zone-Perfect meal. Think of this chapter not as 150 Zone-Perfect meals, but as literally thousands of Zone-Perfect meals.

BREAKFAST

TEXAS-STYLE OMELETTE

Servings: 1 Breakfast Entrée (4 blocks)

Block Size:	Ingredients:
2 Protein	3 ounces lean ground turkey
2 Protein	½ cup egg substitute
1 Carbohydrate	¼ cup canned kidney beans, rinsed and diced*
1 Carbohydrate	½ cup salsa**
1 Carbohydrate	1 cup Zoned Country-Style Chicken Gravy (see page 149)
½ Carbohydrate	1½ cups bean sprouts
½ Carbohydrate	¾ cup red and green bell peppers
4 Fat	1⅓ teaspoons olive oil

Spices:

¼ teaspoon hot sauce

Method:

In a nonstick sauté pan, add the oil, and heat over medium-high heat. In a medium bowl, blend the ground turkey, egg substitute, kidney beans, salsa, and hot sauce. Add egg mixture to heated pan. Let cook until set, then (flip) turn over egg mixture. While omelette is cooking, heat a second nonstick sauté pan. In a small bowl, mix the chicken gravy, bean sprouts, and mixed peppers. Pour into second pan. Cook over medium heat, to blend flavors. When omelette is browned on both sides, place it on a serving dish and top it with the gravy.

*Note: When using canned beans, always rinse them before using.

**Note: Salsa comes with different levels of heat. Choose one that best fits your family's tastes.

SCRAMBLED EGG POCKET WITH MIXED FRUIT SALAD

Servings: 1 Breakfast Entrée (4 blocks)

Block Size:	Ingredients:
3 Protein	¾ cup egg substitute
1 Protein	1 ounce low-fat cheddar cheese, shredded
1 Carbohydrate	½ mini pita pocket
1 Carbohydrate	½ apple, chopped*
1 Carbohydrate	½ pear, chopped
1 Carbohydrate	¾ cup cantaloupe**
4 Fat	4 teaspoons almonds, slivered

Spices:

1 teaspoon chives, chopped
⅛ teaspoon dill
Dash chili powder
Dash celery salt
Black pepper to taste
1 teaspoon lemon juice

Method:
Combine egg substitute, chives, dill, chili powder, celery salt, and pepper. Pour mixture into a microwave-safe 10-ounce dish. Cook in microwave on high (100 percent) setting for 1 to 2½ minutes, until almost set. Push cooked egg portions to center of the dish and continue cooking in 30-second intervals on high setting. When the egg is set, sprinkle with cheese and let stand 2 minutes. Scoop egg mixture into pita pocket. In a medium bowl combine fruit and almonds. Place pita pocket and fruit on a breakfast plate and serve.

*Note: To stop apples from turning brown, dip cut apples in a little lemon juice and water mixture.

**Note:* Depending on the size of the cantaloupe, you may not need all the flesh—store the excess for use in another recipe.*

HERBED OMELETTE

Servings: 1 Breakfast Entrée (4 blocks)

Block Size:	Ingredients:
4 Protein	1 cup egg substitute
½ Carbohydrate	5½ cups alfalfa sprouts
½ Carbohydrate	½ cup onion, chopped
½ Carbohydrate	¾ cup red and green bell peppers
½ Carbohydrate	1½ cups mushrooms, sliced
1 Carbohydrate	½ cup salsa*
1 Carbohydrate	⅓ cup Mandarin orange sections
4 Fat	1⅓ teaspoons olive oil

Spices:

¼ teaspoon garlic, minced
⅛ teaspoon dried oregano
⅛ teaspoon dill
⅛ teaspoon chili powder
⅛ teaspoon dried parsley
⅛ teaspoon Worcestershire sauce
⅛ teaspoon cilantro
Dash lemon herb seasoning

Method:

In a nonstick sauté pan, heat oil over medium-high heat. In a medium bowl, combine the onion, bell peppers, and mushrooms. Add garlic, oregano, dill, chili powder, parsley, Worcestershire sauce, cilantro, and lemon herb seasoning. Spoon vegetable/herb mixture into pan and sauté for 3 minutes, until vegetables soften and herbs are heated. Pour egg substitute into pan, stir to distribute vegetables, and cook until almost set.

Sprinkle sprouts onto half of omelette and fold over. Remove to serving plate. Decorate with orange sections and top omelette with salsa.

Note: Salsa comes with different levels of heat. Choose one that best fits your family's tastes.

YOGURT-TOPPED APPLE

Servings: 1 Breakfast Entrée (4 blocks)

Block Size:	Ingredients:
3 Protein	¾ cup low-fat cottage cheese
1 Protein	½ cup plain low-fat yogurt
1 Carbohydrate	
2 Carbohydrate	1 apple, cored and halved lengthwise*
1 Carbohydrate	1 teaspoon raisins, diced
4 Fat	4 teaspoons almonds, slivered

Spices:

⅛ teaspoon nutmeg
⅛ teaspoon orange zest
⅛ teaspoon cinnamon

Method:
Place apple cut side up in a small microwaveable dish. Spoon raisins into core of apple. Cook the apple in microwave set on high (100 percent) for 4 to 5 minutes. In a small mixing bowl combine yogurt, nutmeg, orange zest, and cinnamon. Place cottage cheese in a serving dish, sprinkled with almonds. When the apple is cooked (slightly soft) place apple on top of cottage cheese, top with yogurt, and serve.

Note: To stop apples from turning brown, dip cut apples in a little lemon juice and water mixture.

COTTAGE CHEESE FRUIT SALAD

Servings: 1 Breakfast Entrée (4 blocks)

Block Size:	Ingredients:
4 Protein	1 cup low-fat cottage cheese
2 Carbohydrate	1 apple, cored and chopped*
1 Carbohydrate	1 teaspoon raisins, chopped
1 Carbohydrate	½ cup pineapple, chopped
4 Fat	4 teaspoons almonds, chopped

Spices:

⅛ teaspoon cinnamon
⅛ teaspoon cilantro
⅛ teaspoon nutmeg

Method:

In a medium serving bowl combine cottage cheese, apple, raisins, pineapple, and almonds. Sprinkle with cinnamon, cilantro, and nutmeg. Serve immediately.

Note: To stop apples from turning brown, dip cut apples in a little lemon juice and water mixture.

POACHED FRUIT WITH CHEESE

Servings: 1 Breakfast Entrée (4 blocks)

Block Size:	Ingredients:
4 Protein	1 cup low-fat cottage cheese
2 Carbohydrate	1 apple, cored and cut in 8 wedges*
1 Carbohydrate	⅓ cup Mandarin orange sections
1 Carbohydrate	½ pear, cut in 3 wedges
4 Fat	4 teaspoons almonds, chopped

Spices:

1 cup water
1-inch piece cinnamon stick
⅛ teaspoon nutmeg

Method:
In medium saucepan bring water, cinnamon, and nutmeg to a boil. Add apple and pear, return to a boil, and cover. Reduce heat to a simmer and cook 5 to 6 minutes. Add orange sections and simmer 1 minute more. Place cottage cheese sprinkled with almonds in a serving bowl. Remove apple and pear with slotted spoon to serving bowl, and place on top of cottage cheese. Serve immediately.

*Note: To stop apples from turning brown, dip cut apples in a little lemon juice and water mixture.

CURRIED ASPARAGUS OMELETTE

Servings: 1 Breakfast Entrée (4 blocks)

Block Size:	Ingredients:
4 Protein	1 cup egg substitute
1 Carbohydrate	½ cup tomato, seeded and chopped
½ Carbohydrate	1½ cups mushrooms, chopped
2 Carbohydrate	2 cups steamed asparagus, 1-inch pieces
½ Carbohydrate	½ cup onion, chopped
4 Fat	1⅓ teaspoons olive oil, divided

Spices:

½ teaspoon garlic, minced
½ to 1 teaspoon curry powder
⅛ teaspoon Worcestershire sauce
1 teaspoon parsley, chopped
⅛ teaspoon turmeric
Salt and pepper to taste

Method:
In a medium nonstick sauté pan, heat half of the oil. Add garlic and cook until lightly browned. Stir in curry powder, Worcestershire sauce, turmeric, and salt and pepper. Cook 1 minute to heat through. Add tomato and mushrooms, asparagus and onion. Cook until softened, about 5 minutes. Cover and remove from heat. In a second nonstick sauté pan, heat remaining oil. Pour egg substitute into second sauté pan and cook until set. Place omelette on serving plate and spoon asparagus mixture onto half of omelette and fold other half over. Sprinkle with parsley and serve immediately.

ORIENTAL VEGETABLE OMELETTE

Servings: 1 Breakfast Entrée (4 blocks)

Block Size:	Ingredients:
4 Protein	1 cup egg substitute
½ Carbohydrate	½ cup scallions, thinly sliced diagonally
1 Carbohydrate	1 cup canned mushrooms, sliced
½ Carbohydrate	2¼ cups red and green bell peppers
1 Carbohydrate	¼ cup chickpeas
1 Carbohydrate	3 cups bean sprouts
4 Fat	1⅓ teaspoons olive oil, divided

Spices:

½ teaspoon garlic, minced
3 tablespoons cider vinegar
½ teaspoon gingerroot, grated*
1 tablespoon soy sauce
⅛ teaspoon Worcestershire sauce

Method:

In large nonstick sauté pan, heat half of the oil. Stir-fry scallions for 1 minute over medium-high heat. Add mushrooms and cook another 2 minutes, then add peppers, chickpeas, sprouts, garlic, vinegar, ginger, soy sauce, and Worcestershire sauce. Cook 3 to 5 minutes or until bean sprouts are tender. In a second large nonstick sauté pan, heat remaining oil on medium-high heat. Pour in egg substitute. As it cooks, push cooked portions toward center of pan with a spatula. When eggs are set, remove omelette to warmed serving plate and place filling from first pan into one side of omelette and fold other side and serve.

*Note: When a recipe calls for fresh ginger root (available in most grocery stores or Asian markets), it is not advisable to substitute ground ginger. The flavors are very different.

OMELETTE ROCKEFELLER

Servings: 1 Breakfast Entrée (4 blocks)

Block Size:	Ingredients:
4 Protein	1 cup egg substitute
½ Carbohydrate	2 cups watercress, chopped
½ Carbohydrate	½ cup onion, chopped
½ Carbohydrate	3 cups raw spinach*
1 Carbohydrate	1 cup canned mushrooms, chopped
½ Carbohydrate	1½ cups bean sprouts
1 Carbohydrate	½ cup salsa**
3 Fat	1 teaspoon olive oil, divided
1 Fat	1 teaspoon almonds, finely chopped

Spices:

½ teaspoon garlic, minced, divided
⅛ teaspoon cayenne pepper
⅛ teaspoon nutmeg
⅛ teaspoon celery salt
1 tablespoon balsamic vinegar
Salt and pepper to taste

Method:
In a medium nonstick sauté pan, heat oil. Mix egg substitute, ¼ teaspoon garlic, salt and pepper. Pour into sauté pan and cook until set. In a small nonstick saucepan heat onion, salsa, ¼ teaspoon garlic, cayenne, nutmeg, celery salt, vinegar, and salt and pepper. Bring to boil, reduce heat, cover and gently simmer 2 to 3 minutes. On half of serving plate combine watercress, spinach, mushrooms, and sprouts. Place omelette on the other side, top all with sauce, sprinkle with almonds, and serve.

*Note: Fresh spinach needs to be cleaned very well, because of its tendency

to have sand on it, so be sure to soak spinach in water to remove any sand or dirt before using.

**Note: Salsa comes with different levels of heat. Choose one that best fits your taste.

FLORENTINE FILLED CREPES

Servings: 1 Breakfast Entrée (4 blocks)

Block Size:	Ingredients:
4 Protein	1 cup egg substitute
1 Carbohydrate	3 cups mushrooms, sliced
½ Carbohydrate	½ cup onion, chopped
½ Carbohydrate	3 cups fresh spinach, torn*
1 Carbohydrate	2 cups alfalfa sprouts
1 Carbohydrate	1 kiwi fruit, peeled and sliced
4 Fat	1⅓ teaspoons olive oil, divided

Spices:

⅛ teaspoon celery salt
⅛ teaspoon nutmeg
⅛ teaspoon cinnamon
4 tablespoons balsamic vinegar
Salt and pepper to taste

Method:
In a large nonstick sauté pan, heat ⅔ teaspoon oil. Combine egg substitute, celery salt, nutmeg, and cinnamon. Pour into sauté pan. When browned on one side flip over with spatula and brown the other side. Heat remaining oil in a second nonstick sauté pan, over a medium-high heat. When heated, add mushrooms and onion. Cook for 3 to 5 minutes, then add balsamic vinegar, spinach, and sprouts. Continue cook-

ing until spinach is just wilted. Place omelette onto serving plate. Spoon vegetable mixture onto omelette and fold over. Decorate with kiwi fruit and serve.

Note: Fresh spinach needs to be cleaned very well, because of its tendency to have sand on it, so be sure to soak spinach in water to remove any sand or dirt before using.

SPICY SHRIMP AND MUSHROOM OMELETTE

Servings: 1 Breakfast Entrée (4 blocks)

Block Size:	Ingredients:
1 Protein	1½ ounces shrimp, chopped
3 Protein	¾ cup egg substitute
1 Carbohydrate	1 cup onion, chopped
1 Carbohydrate	3 cups mushrooms, chopped
1 Carbohydrate	1 kiwi fruit, peeled and sliced
1 Carbohydrate	1 cup asparagus spears
4 Fat	1⅓ teaspoons olive oil

Spices:

⅛ teaspoon garlic, minced
¼ teaspoon dried parsley, chopped
⅛ teaspoon dry mustard
⅛ teaspoon dried basil
⅛ teaspoon cayenne pepper
⅛ teaspoon turmeric
Salt and pepper to taste

Method:

In a medium nonstick sauté pan, heat oil. Add asparagus and spices to sauté pan and cook for 1 minute, then add onion and mushrooms. Cook for 3 to 5 minutes or until vegetables are tender. Remove vegetables and keep warm. Place shrimp in sauté pan and cook for 1 minute. Pour egg substitute into sauté pan. Stir to make sure shrimp is distributed throughout the egg. Cook on medium-high heat until omelette is almost set. Remove omelette to serving plate. Spoon onion/mushroom mixture onto omelette and fold over. Decorate omelette with kiwi slices and serve.

FRUITY-NUT COTTAGE CHEESE WITH RASPBERRY SAUCE

Servings: 1 Breakfast Entrée (4 blocks)

Block Size:	Ingredients:
4 Protein	1 cup low-fat cottage cheese
½ Carbohydrate	¼ cup fresh blueberries
1 Carbohydrate	½ cup peaches, diced
½ Carbohydrate	¾ cup cantaloupe, diced
½ Carbohydrate	¼ cup grapes
1½ Carbohydrate	1½ cups raspberries
4 Fat	4 macadamia nuts, chopped

Method:

This recipe requires a blender or food processor. Mound cottage cheese in center of serving plate. Arrange blueberries, peaches, cantaloupe, and grapes around cottage cheese. Place raspberries in blender and puree. Pour pureed raspberries over cottage cheese and fruit, then sprinkle with nuts and serve.

JAPANESE-STYLE CHICKEN AND SPINACH OMELETTE

Servings: 1 Breakfast Entrée (4 blocks)

Block Size:	Ingredients:
2 Protein	½ cup egg substitute
2 Protein	2 ounces chicken tenderloins, diced
1 Carbohydrate	6 cups spinach*
1 Carbohydrate	3 cups mushrooms, sliced
1 Carbohydrate	3 cups bean sprouts
1 Carbohydrate	1 cup onion, diced
4 Fat	1⅓ teaspoons olive oil, divided

Spices:

1 tablespoon soy sauce
¼ teaspoon Worcestershire sauce
2 tablespoons balsamic vinegar
⅛ teaspoon chili powder
⅛ teaspoon cayenne pepper
⅛ teaspoon celery salt

Method:

Heat 1 teaspoon oil in a medium nonstick sauté pan. Sauté chicken and onion until lightly browned. Add spinach, mushrooms, and bean sprouts. Cook 3 to 5 minutes. Add remaining oil to another sauté pan. In a small bowl stir soy sauce, Worcestershire sauce, balsamic vinegar, and seasonings into egg substitute, then pour into sauté pan. Cook until almost set. Spoon vegetables onto half of omelette. Fold over and cook 1 additional minute. Place omelette on serving plate and serve.

*Note: Fresh spinach needs to be cleaned very well, because of its tendency to have sand on it, so be sure to soak spinach in water to remove any sand or dirt before using.

TOMATO OMELETTE WITH SAUTÉED PEPPER AND CHEESE

Servings: 1 Breakfast Entrée (4 blocks)

Block Size:	Ingredients:
3 Protein	¾ cup egg substitute
1 Protein	1 ounce shredded low-fat cheddar cheese
¾ Carbohydrate	¾ cup canned mushrooms, chopped
1 Carbohydrate	2¼ cups bell peppers, chopped
½ Carbohydrate	½ cup pearl onions, frozen
1 Carbohydrate	1¼ cups tomato, seeded and diced
½ Carbohydrate	¼ cup salsa*
¼ Carbohydrate	1 teaspoon cornstarch
4 Fat	1⅓ teaspoons olive oil, divided

Spices:

½ teaspoon garlic, minced
⅛ teaspoon celery salt
¼ teaspoon Worcestershire sauce
1 tablespoon cider vinegar
Salt and pepper to taste

Method:

In a medium nonstick sauté pan heat ⅔ teaspoon oil. Add mushrooms and sauté for 3 minutes. Stir in peppers and cook an additional 3 minutes. Add onions, tomatoes, salsa, and cornstarch to form a sauce. (Mix cornstarch with a little water to dissolve it before adding to pan.) Heat remaining oil in a second sauté pan. In a small bowl combine egg substitute, garlic, celery salt, Worcestershire sauce, cider vinegar, and salt and pepper. Pour into second sauté pan. Cook until almost set. Spoon mushroom mixture onto half of omelette. Fold over and cook for an additional 3 to 5 minutes. Lift with spatula onto serving dish. Top with shredded cheese and serve.

Note: Salsa comes with different levels of heat. Choose one that best fits your family's tastes.

SOUTHWESTERN HAM OMELETTE WITH TACO CHEESE

Servings: 1 Breakfast Entrée (4 blocks)

Block Size:	Ingredients:
2 Protein	½ cup egg substitute
1 Protein	1 ounce low-fat taco-style cheese, shredded
1 Protein	1½ ounces deli-style ham, diced
½ Carbohydrate	½ cup onion, diced
1 Carbohydrate	2¼ cups peppers, chopped
1 Carbohydrate	1¼ cups tomatoes, chopped
½ Carbohydrate	¼ cup salsa*
½ Carbohydrate	¼ cup cooked kidney beans, rinsed
½ Carbohydrate	2 teaspoons cornstarch
4 Fat	1⅓ teaspoons olive oil, divided

Spices:

½ teaspoon garlic, minced
⅛ teaspoon chili powder
1 tablespoon apple cider
½ teaspoon cilantro, chopped
⅛ teaspoon celery salt
Salt and pepper to taste

Method:

In a medium nonstick sauté pan, heat ⅔ teaspoon of oil. Combine onion, peppers, tomato, salsa, kidney beans, cornstarch, and seasonings. (Mix cornstarch with a little water to dissolve it before adding to pan.) Cook for 5 to 8 minutes, stirring occasionally. In a second sauté pan, heat remaining oil. Using a medium bowl, blend egg substitute, ham, and salt and pepper. Pour into pan and stir to distribute ham evenly. Cook until set. Flip omelette over with spatula and cook another 2 minutes. Place omelette on serving plate and spoon pepper mixture onto half of omelette. Fold omelette over and sprinkle with cheese and serve.

Note: Salsa comes with different levels of heat. Choose one that best fits your taste. We used a medium salsa here.

ASPARAGUS OMELETTE WITH CHEESE

Servings: 1 Breakfast Entrée (4 blocks)

Block Size:	Ingredients:
3 Protein	¾ cup egg substitute
1 Protein	1 ounce shredded low-fat cheese
1 Carbohydrate	1 cup pearl onions, frozen
1 Carbohydrate	1¼ cups tomatoes, chopped
1 Carbohydrate	¼ cup cooked kidney beans, rinsed and chopped
1 Carbohydrate	1 cup asparagus spears, chopped
4 Fat	1⅓ teaspoons olive oil, divided

Spices:

1 teaspoon garlic, minced
⅛ teaspoon celery salt
⅛ teaspoon lemon herb seasoning
⅛ teaspoon chili powder
½ teaspoon balsamic vinegar
⅛ teaspoon Worcestershire sauce
Salt and pepper to taste

Method:

In a medium nonstick sauté pan heat, ⅔ teaspoon oil. Sauté onion, tomato, beans, asparagus, and seasonings for 5 to 7 minutes. Heat remaining oil in second sauté pan. Pour in egg substitute, spread around pan, and lightly season with salt and pepper. When set, spoon mixture onto half of omelette. Fold over and remove to serving plate. Top with cheese and serve.

BLUEBERRY COTTAGE CHEESE

Servings: 1 Breakfast Entrée (4 blocks)

Block Size:	Ingredients:
3 Protein	¾ cup low-fat cottage cheese
1 Protein and	½ cup plain low-fat yogurt
1 Carbohydrate	
1 Carbohydrate	⅓ cup unsweetened applesauce
2 Carbohydrate	1 cup blueberries, fresh or frozen
4 Fat	4 teaspoons slivered almonds

Spices:

¼ teaspoon cinnamon
¼ teaspoon nutmeg

Method:

This recipe requires a blender or food processor. Place blueberries and applesauce, nutmeg and cinnamon in a blender and pulse 2 or 3 times. In a medium bowl, combine blueberry mixture, yogurt, and cottage cheese. Sprinkle with almonds and serve.

STEAK WITH MORNING VEGETABLE MEDLEY

Servings: 1 Breakfast Entrée (4 blocks)

Block Size:	Ingredients:
4 Protein	4 ounces sirloin steak, ¾ inch thick
1 Carbohydrate	1¼ cups tomatoes, chopped
1 Carbohydrate	1 cup pearl onions, frozen
1 Carbohydrate	1 cup green beans
½ Carbohydrate	3 cups fresh spinach*
½ Carbohydrate	¼ cup cooked kidney beans
4 Fat	1⅓ teaspoons olive oil, divided

Spices:

2 teaspoons garlic, minced
¼ teaspoon Worcestershire sauce
⅛ teaspoon celery salt
1 tablespoon cider vinegar
1 teaspoon parsley, chopped
Salt and pepper to taste

Method:

In a medium nonstick sauté pan, heat ⅔ teaspoon oil. Combine all vegetables and seasonings and sauté 5 to 7 minutes until crisp-tender. In a second sauté pan, heat remaining oil and sauté steak until cooked to the desired degree. Place steak on one side of serving dish and vegetables on the other.

Note: Fresh spinach needs to be cleaned very well, because of its tendency to have sand in it, so be sure to soak spinach in water to remove any sand or dirt before using.

WINTER FRUIT COMPOTE

Servings: 1 Breakfast Entrée (4 blocks)

Block Size:	Ingredients:
4 Protein	1 cup low-fat cottage cheese
1 Carbohydrate	½ grapefruit, in sections
1 Carbohydrate	⅓ cup Mandarin orange sections
2 Carbohydrate	1 Granny Smith apple, cored and chopped
4 Fat	4 teaspoons almonds, slivered and toasted

Spices:
⅛ teaspoon cinnamon
⅛ teaspoon nutmeg
Paprika to taste

Method:
In small mixing bowl combine cottage cheese with cinnamon and nutmeg. Mound onto serving dish. Arrange grapefruit and orange sections around cheese. Combine almonds and apple pieces and spoon over cheese. Sprinkle paprika over cheese and serve.

CHICKEN AND CHICKPEA HASH

Servings: 1 Breakfast Entrée (4 blocks)

Block Size:	Ingredients:
4 Protein	6 ounces ground chicken
½ Carbohydrate	1½ cups mushrooms, diced
½ Carbohydrate	½ cup onion, diced
1 Carbohydrate	⅓ cup boiled potato, mashed (without butter or milk)
2 Carbohydrate	½ cup cooked chickpeas, mashed
4 Fat	1⅓ teaspoons olive oil

Spices:

⅛ teaspoon Worcestershire sauce
⅛ teaspoon lemon herb seasoning
⅛ teaspoon chili powder
Paprika for garnish
Parsley for garnish

Method:

In a medium nonstick sauté pan, heat oil. Sauté chicken, onion, and mushrooms until chicken is cooked. Add remaining ingredients (except paprika and parsley) and cook on medium-high heat until browned, about 3 to 5 minutes. Place on a heated serving dish. Garnish with parsley and paprika.

MANDARIN ORANGE COTTAGE CHEESE SCRAMBLE

Servings: 1 Breakfast Entrée (4 blocks)

Block Size:	Ingredients:
1 Protein	¼ cup low-fat cottage cheese
3 Protein	¾ cup egg substitute
½ Carbohydrate	1½ cups mushrooms, sliced
½ Carbohydrate	½ cup onion, chopped
1 Carbohydrate	2¼ cups mixed peppers, cut in half and sliced*
1 Carbohydrate	1 cup snow peas, julienned
1 Carbohydrate	⅓ cup Mandarin orange sections
4 Fat	1⅓ teaspoons olive oil

Spices:

1 tablespoon balsamic vinegar
¼ teaspoon Worcestershire sauce
⅛ teaspoon celery salt
¼ teaspoon dried dill
¼ teaspoon lemon herb seasoning

Method:

Heat oil in a medium nonstick sauté pan. Sauté mushrooms, onion, peppers, vinegar, Worcestershire sauce, celery salt, and dill. Cook until the vegetables are crisp-tender, about 5 to 7 minutes. Then pour in the egg substitute and snow peas. Cook, stirring, until set. Remove from heat and stir in cottage cheese and mandarin orange sections. Sprinkle on lemon herb seasoning and serve.

*Note: Equal portions of red, yellow, and green peppers.

ITALIAN SAUSAGE AND APPLE COMPOTE

Servings: 1 Breakfast Entrée (4 blocks)

Block Size:	Ingredients:
4 Protein	8 links Italian soy sausages, chopped
2 Carbohydrate	1 Granny Smith apple, cored and chopped
2 Carbohydrate	⅔ cup unsweetened applesauce
4 Fat	1⅓ teaspoons olive oil

Spices:

1 tablespoon balsamic vinegar
2 tablespoons cider vinegar
⅛ teaspoon celery salt
⅓ cup water
⅛ teaspoon cinnamon

Method:

Heat oil in a medium nonstick sauté pan. Sauté sausage with celery salt and vinegars. Cook until sausage is browned. Add apple and cook until it begins to soften but is still crunchy. Add applesauce, cinnamon, and water; reduce heat, and simmer 2 to 3 minutes. Spoon into bowl and serve.

BERRY OMELETTE

Servings: 1 Breakfast Entrée (4 blocks)

Block Size:	Ingredients:
4 Protein	1 cup egg substitute
1 Carbohydrate	½ nectarine, pitted and chopped
1 Carbohydrate	½ cup blueberries
½ Carbohydrate	½ cup raspberries
½ Carbohydrate	¼ cup seedless grapes
1 Carbohydrate	⅓ cup applesauce
4 Fat	1⅓ teaspoons olive oil

Spices:

⅛ teaspoon celery salt

⅓ cup water

⅛ teaspoon cinnamon

Salt and pepper to taste

Method:

Heat oil in medium nonstick sauté pan. Season egg substitute and pour into pan. Cook until set and flip over with a spatula. Cook an additional minute. Fold omelette onto serving dish and keep warm. Combine fruits, water, and cinnamon in a saucepan, heat until hot, then spoon over omelette and serve.

CILANTRO EGG SALAD

Servings: 1 Breakfast Entrée (4 blocks)

Block Size:	Ingredients:
4 Protein	1 cup egg substitute
¼ Carbohydrate	¼ cup celery, minced
½ Carbohydrate	½ cup canned mushrooms, diced
¼ Carbohydrate	¼ cup onion, chopped
1 Carbohydrate	¼ cup kidney beans
½ Carbohydrate	2 cups lettuce
½ Carbohydrate	2 cups cucumber, peeled and sliced
1 Carbohydrate	1¼ cups tomatoes, diced
4 Fat	4 teaspoons reduced-fat mayonnaise

Spices:

⅛ teaspoon dry mustard
½ teaspoon garlic, minced
⅛ teaspoon cilantro
Salt and pepper to taste

Method:
Pour egg substitute into a 10-ounce microwave-safe dish and cook on high (100 percent) setting for 1 to 2½ minutes, or until set, push cooked egg portions to center of the dish and continue cooking in 30-second intervals on high setting. When done, cool and dice cooked egg substitute. In a small bowl, blend mayonnaise and seasonings. Combine cooked egg substitute with the other ingredients in a medium bowl and toss to coat with mayonnaise and serve.

LUNCH

MEDITERRANEAN BEEF SALAD

Servings: 1 Lunch Entrée (4 blocks)

Block Size:	Ingredients:
4 Protein	4 ounces beef eye of round, ⅛-inch slices, cut in ½-inch pieces
1 Carbohydrate	2¼ cups red and green pepper strips
1 Carbohydrate	1 cup onion, chopped
1 Carbohydrate	1 cup Zoned Mushroom Sauce (see page 148)
1 Carbohydrate	3 cups garden salad mix (lettuce and shredded red cabbage)
4 Fat	1⅓ teaspoons olive oil

Spices:

⅛ teaspoon Worcestershire sauce
⅛ teaspoon red wine
Salt and pepper to taste

Method:
In a nonstick sauté pan, add oil, beef, peppers, onion, Worcestershire sauce, and red wine. Cook until beef is browned and pepper and onions are tender, then add Zoned Mushroom Sauce. Cover and simmer for 5 minutes until mixture is hot, stirring occasionally to blend flavors. On a large oval plate, arrange garden salad mix. Spoon beef and vegetable mixture into the center of plate, on top of garden salad. Sprinkle with salt and pepper and serve immediately.

GERMAN TURKEY SALAD

Servings: 1 Lunch Entrée (4 blocks)

Block Size:	Ingredients:
4 Protein	6 ounces ground turkey
½ Carbohydrate	¾ cup broccoli florets
½ Carbohydrate	1 cup cauliflower florets
1 Carbohydrate	2¼ cups bell pepper strips*
1 Carbohydrate	3 cups shredded cabbage (or coleslaw mix)
1 Carbohydrate	½ cup Zoned French Dressing (see page 157)
4 Fat	1⅓ teaspoons olive oil

Spices:

⅛ teaspoon balsamic vinegar
⅛ teaspoon Worcestershire sauce
1 teaspoon minced garlic
Salt and pepper to taste

Method:

In a nonstick sauté pan, add oil, ground turkey, broccoli, cauliflower, bell pepper strips, balsamic vinegar, Worcestershire sauce, and garlic. Cook until ground turkey is browned and vegetables are tender, then add Zoned French Dressing. Cover and simmer for 5 minutes until mixture is hot, stirring occasionally to blend flavors. On a large oval plate arrange shredded cabbage. Spoon ground turkey and vegetable mixture into the center of plate, on top of the shredded cabbage. Sprinkle with salt and pepper and serve immediately.

Note: Equal portions of red, yellow, and green peppers.

BARBECUE CHICKEN SALAD

Servings: 1 Lunch Entrée (4 blocks)

Block Size:	Ingredients:
4 Protein	4 ounces chicken tenderloin, diced (or skinless chicken breast)
1 Carbohydrate	2¼ cups bell pepper strips
1 Carbohydrate	1 cup onions, diced
1 Carbohydrate	½ cup Zoned Barbecue Sauce (see page 154)
½ Carbohydrate	1½ cups garden salad mix (lettuce and shredded red cabbage)
½ Carbohydrate	1½ cups shredded cabbage (or coleslaw mix)
4 Fat	1⅓ teaspoons olive oil

Spices:

⅛ teaspoon cider vinegar
⅛ teaspoon Worcestershire sauce
1 teaspoon minced garlic
Salt and pepper to taste

Method:

In a nonstick sauté pan, add oil, chicken tenderloins, pepper, onion, vinegar, Worcestershire sauce, and garlic. Cook until chicken is browned and vegetables are tender, then add Zoned Barbecue Sauce. Cover and simmer for 5 minutes until mixture is hot, stirring occasionally to blend flavors. Blend together garden salad mix and shredded cabbage, then place blended salad-cabbage mixture on a large oval plate. Spoon chicken and vegetable mixture into the center of plate on top of salad-cabbage mixture. Sprinkle with salt and pepper and serve immediately.

HERBED SEAFOOD SALAD

Servings: 1 Lunch Entrée (4 blocks)

Block Size:	Ingredients:
2 Protein	3 ounces clams
2 Protein	3 ounces bay scallops
1 Carbohydrate	½ cup Zoned Herb Dressing (see page 156)
½ Carbohydrate	1½ cups shredded cabbage
½ Carbohydrate	1½ cups garden salad mix (lettuce and shredded red cabbage)
½ Carbohydrate	2 cups cucumber, peeled, seeded, and roughly chopped
1 Carbohydrate	2¼ cups bell pepper strips
½ Carbohydrate	½ cup onion, chopped
4 Fat	1⅓ teaspoons olive oil

Spices:

⅛ teaspoon Worcestershire sauce
1 teaspoon dry mustard
⅛ teaspoon white wine

Method:
Heat oil in medium nonstick sauté pan. Add clams, scallops, pepper strips, onion, Worcestershire sauce, mustard, and wine. Sauté until cooked through; add Zoned Herb Dressing. Simmer for 3 to 5 minutes. Combine vegetables in medium bowl. Pour seafood mixture over vegetables.

DILLED CHICKEN GARDEN SALAD

Servings: 1 Lunch Entrée (4 blocks)

Block Size:	Ingredients:
4 Protein	4 ounces chicken tenderloin
1 Carbohydrate	½ cup Zoned Herb Dressing (see page 156)
1 Carbohydrate	1 cup onion, chopped
½ Carbohydrate	2 cups romaine lettuce, torn
½ Carbohydrate	1½ cups garden salad mix (lettuce and shredded red cabbage)
1 Carbohydrate	3 cups mushrooms, sliced
4 Fat	1⅓ teaspoons olive oil

Spices:

⅛ teaspoon Worcestershire sauce
¼ teaspoon lemon herb seasoning
1 tablespoon cider vinegar
1 teaspoon dried dill weed
Salt and pepper to taste

Method:

Heat oil in medium nonstick sauté pan. Add chicken, mushrooms, onion, Worcestershire sauce, lemon and herb seasoning, cider vinegar, dill, and salt and pepper. Sauté until cooked through. Drain off excess liquid. Stir in Zoned Herb Dressing and simmer 3 to 5 minutes. Combine romaine and salad mix in a medium bowl. Top with chicken mixture and serve.

FLORENTINE CRAB SALAD

Servings: 1 Lunch Entrée (4 blocks)

Block Size:	Ingredients:
4 Protein	6 ounces canned crabmeat
½ Carbohydrate	½ cup scallions, sliced (white and green parts)
½ Carbohydrate	1½ cups mushrooms, sliced
1 Carbohydrate	¼ cup cooked kidney beans, rinsed
½ Carbohydrate	2 cups raw spinach, stems removed
½ Carbohydrate	1½ cups shredded cabbage (or coleslaw mix)
1 Carbohydrate	½ cup Zoned Herb Dressing (see page 156)
4 Fat	1⅓ teaspoons olive oil

Spices:

1 tablespoon balsamic vinegar
⅛ teaspoon Worcestershire sauce
⅛ teaspoon celery salt
½ teaspoon garlic, minced
2 teaspoons white Zinfandel wine
⅛ teaspoon chili powder
Pepper to taste

Method:
Heat oil in a medium nonstick sauté pan. Add crab, scallions, mushrooms, kidney beans, vinegar, Worcestershire sauce, celery salt, garlic, wine, chili powder, and pepper. Sauté until cooked through. Stir in Zoned Herb Dressing. Simmer 3 to 5 minutes. In a medium bowl combine spinach and cabbage. Top with crab mixture and serve.

TUNA SALAD WITH CABBAGE

Servings: 1 Lunch Entrée (4 blocks)

Block Size:	Ingredients:
4 Protein	4 ounces albacore tuna in water
1 Carbohydrate	½ cup Zoned French Dressing (see page 157)
½ Carbohydrate	1½ cups shredded cabbage (or coleslaw mix)
½ Carbohydrate	1½ cups garden salad mix (lettuce and shredded red cabbage)
1 Carbohydrate	1¼ cups tomato, diced
½ Carbohydrate	1¼ cups celery, chopped
¼ Carbohydrate	¼ cup asparagus, chopped
¼ Carbohydrate	¼ cup scallion, chopped (white and green parts)
2 Fat	6 olives, chopped coarsely
2 Fat	⅔ teaspoon olive oil

Spices:

⅛ teaspoon lemon herb seasoning
⅛ teaspoon chili powder
1 tablespoon cider vinegar

Method:
Combine tuna, tomato, celery, asparagus, scallion, olives, oil, Zoned French Dressing, lemon herb seasoning, chili powder, and vinegar. Arrange garden salad mix and shredded cabbage on a serving plate. Place tuna mixture on top of greens and serve.

HERBED STIR-FRY SCALLOPS WITH MIXED VEGETABLES

Servings: 1 Lunch Entrée (4 blocks)

Block Size:	Ingredients:
4 Protein	6 ounces baby bay scallops
½ Carbohydrate	¾ cup broccoli florets
¾ Carbohydrate	¾ cup green beans
¾ Carbohydrate	¾ cup pearl onions, frozen
½ Carbohydrate	1⅛ cup red pepper strips
½ Carbohydrate	1½ cups mushrooms, sliced
1 Carbohydrate	½ cup Zoned Herb Dressing* (see page 156)
4 Fat	1⅓ teaspoons olive oil, divided

Spices:

2 tablespoons lemon- or lime-flavored spring water

Method:

In a nonstick sauté pan, place ⅔ teaspoon oil, flavored water, and scallops. Cook until scallops are done. While the scallops are cooking over medium heat, in another sauté pan, place vegetables, ⅔ teaspoon oil, and Zoned Herb Dressing. Heat vegetables until entire mixture is hot, then add scallops. Cook for 3 to 4 minutes until entire stir-fry is hot and vegetables and dressing have coated scallops. Spoon onto a lunch dish and serve immediately.

*Note: All the seasonings you need for this dish are in the Zoned Herb Dressing.

SAUTÉED SCALLOPS WITH ARTICHOKE HEARTS

Servings: 1 Lunch Entrée (4 blocks)

Block Size:	Ingredients:
4 Protein	6 ounces baby bay scallops
2 Carbohydrate	6 small artichoke hearts, canned*
1 Carbohydrate	½ cup salsa**
1 Carbohydrate	1 cup Zoned Mushroom Sauce (see page 148)
4 Fat	1⅓ teaspoons olive oil

Spices:

⅛ teaspoon Worcestershire sauce

Method:

Cut artichoke hearts into pieces. Combine with oil and Worcestershire sauce in heated nonstick sauté pan. Heat for 2 to 3 minutes. Add scallops and remaining ingredients and cook on high until the scallops are cooked through.

*Note: 3 small artichoke hearts equal 1 medium artichoke.

**Note: We used a medium-heat salsa, but you can adjust the strength to your family's taste.

SAUTÉED SCALLOPS WITH SPICED PEPPERS AND MUSHROOMS

Servings: 1 Lunch Entrée (4 blocks)

Block Size:	Ingredients:
4 Protein	6 ounces bay scallops
1 Carbohydrate	2¼ cups red and green pepper strips
1 Carbohydrate	¼ cup canned kidney beans, rinsed
1 Carbohydrate	½ cup salsa*
½ Carbohydrate	1½ cups mushrooms, sliced
½ Carbohydrate	2 teaspoons cornstarch
4 Fat	1⅓ teaspoons olive oil

Spices:

1 tablespoon balsamic vinegar
⅛ teaspoon chili powder
⅛ teaspoon hot pepper sauce
⅛ teaspoon ground red pepper

Method:

Heat oil in a nonstick sauté pan and add peppers and salsa. Stir-fry 2 to 3 minutes. Add mushrooms, scallops, kidney beans, spices, and cornstarch. (Mix cornstarch with a little water to dissolve it before adding to pan.) Stir-fry until scallops are cooked through. Just before dish is cooked, add vinegar. Stir and serve.

*Note: We used a medium-heat salsa, but you can adjust the strength to your family's tastes.

FLORENTINE TURKEY SALAD

Servings: 1 Lunch Entrée (4 blocks)

Block Size:	Ingredients:
4 Protein	6 ounces lean ground turkey
½ Carbohydrate	3 cups spinach, chopped*
1 Carbohydrate	½ cup Zoned French Dressing (see page 157)
1½ Carbohydrate	¾ cup salsa**
½ Carbohydrate	1½ cups cabbage, shredded (or coleslaw mix)
½ Carbohydrate	½ cup onion, chopped
4 Fat	1⅓ teaspoons olive oil

Spices:

1 tablespoon cider vinegar
⅛ teaspoon Worcestershire sauce
⅛ teaspoon celery salt
⅛ teaspoon chili powder

Method:

Heat oil in a medium nonstick sauté pan. Add turkey, salsa, onion, vinegar, Worcestershire sauce, celery salt, and chili powder. When turkey is cooked, add Zoned French Dressing. Sauté 3 to 5 minutes. In a medium bowl combine spinach and cabbage. Top with turkey mixture and serve.

*Note: Fresh spinach needs to be cleaned very well, because of sand, so be sure to soak spinach in water to remove any sand or dirt before using.

**Note: We used a medium-heat salsa, but you can adjust the strength to your family's tastes.

CALIFORNIA-STYLE TACOBURGER

Servings: 1 Lunch Entrée (4 blocks)

Block Size:	Ingredients:
4 Protein	6 ounces lean ground turkey
½ Carbohydrate	5½ cups bean sprouts
½ Carbohydrate	1 cup red and green pepper strips
1 Carbohydrate	½ cup salsa*
1 Carbohydrate	½ mini pita pocket (6-inch)
1 Carbohydrate	¼ cup canned kidney beans, rinsed
2 Fat	2 teaspoons almonds, slivered
2 Fat	6 olives, sliced

Spices:

½ teaspoon garlic, minced
¼ teaspoon chili powder, divided
⅛ teaspoon Worcestershire sauce
⅛ teaspoon celery salt
⅛ teaspoon cider vinegar

Method:
Combine the turkey, ⅛ teaspoon chili powder, Worcestershire sauce and 1 cup sprouts and form into patty and bake in a 425-degree Fahrenheit oven for 15 minutes. Mix peppers, salsa, kidney beans, 4½ cups sprouts, and remaining spices. Cook for several minutes, then add vinegar. Add olives and almonds. Stir to blend and heat through. When heated, stuff mini pita with burger and place vegetable mixture on plate and serve.

*Note: We used a medium-heat salsa, but you can adjust the strength to your family's tastes.

ORIENTAL TURKEY WITH SNOW PEAS

Servings: 1 Lunch Entrée (4 blocks)

Block Size:	Ingredients:
4 Protein	6 ounces lean ground turkey
1 Carbohydrate	¾ cup Zoned Espagnol (Brown) Sauce (see page 155)
½ Carbohydrate	5½ cups alfalfa sprouts
1 Carbohydrate	2¼ cups bell pepper strips
½ Carbohydrate	½ cup snow peas
½ Carbohydrate	½ cup pearl onions, frozen
½ Carbohydrate	¾ cup broccoli florets
4 Fat	1⅓ teaspoons olive oil, divided

Spices:

1 teaspoon soy sauce
1 teaspoon Worcestershire sauce
1 tablespoons balsamic vinegar

Method:

In nonstick sauté pan heat ⅔ teaspoon of the olive oil and cook the turkey (breaking it up as it cooks) and alfalfa sprouts. In second nonstick sauté pan, heat remaining olive oil. Sauté peppers, snow peas, onions, broccoli, soy sauce, Worcestershire sauce, and vinegar. Cook until tender, then add Zoned Espagnol Sauce. Blend turkey mixture with vegetables and serve.

STIR-FRY BEEF WITH GREEN BEANS

Servings: 1 Lunch Entrée (4 blocks)

Block Size:	Ingredients:
4 Protein	4 ounces lean beef, small cubes
3 Carbohydrate	3 cups green beans
1 Carbohydrate	½ cup Zoned Tarragon Mustard Sauce (see page 160)
4 Fat	1⅓ teaspoons olive oil, divided

Spices:

¼ teaspoon Worcestershire sauce
½ teaspoon cider vinegar
⅛ teaspoon chili powder
⅛ teaspoon celery salt
⅛ teaspoon tarragon

Method:

Heat ⅔ teaspoon oil in a medium nonstick sauté pan. Add beef and sauté until cooked through. Stir in Zoned Tarragon Mustard Sauce and simmer for 3 to 5 minutes. In second sauté pan, heat remaining oil and sauté green beans, Worcestershire sauce, vinegar, chili powder, celery salt, and tarragon. Cook until beans are crisp-tender, about 5 minutes. Place beans on serving dish and either top with beef mixture or spoon it beside beans.

BEEF ITALIANO

Servings: 1 Lunch Entrée (4 blocks)

Block Size:	Ingredients:
4 Protein	4 ounces lean beef, small cubes
1 Carbohydrate	½ cup Zoned Italian Sauce (see page 150)
1 Carbohydrate	1 cup Italian-style green beans
1 Carbohydrate	2¼ cups red and green pepper strips
½ Carbohydrate	½ cup onion, diced
½ Carbohydrate	¼ cup salsa*
4 Fat	1⅓ teaspoons olive oil, divided

Spices:

½ teaspoon parsley flakes
½ teaspoon Worcestershire sauce
⅛ teaspoon celery salt
⅛ teaspoon lemon herb seasoning
⅛ teaspoon dried oregano

Method:

Heat ⅔ teaspoon oil in a medium nonstick sauté pan. Add beef and sauté until cooked. Add Zoned Italian Sauce and simmer for 3 to 5 minutes. In second nonstick sauté pan, heat remaining oil. Sauté the green beans, pepper strips, onion, salsa, parsley, Worcestershire sauce, celery salt, lemon herb seasoning, and oregano. Cook until crisp-tender, about 5 minutes. Spoon vegetables onto serving dish and top with beef mixture.

*Note: We used a medium-heat salsa. Use whatever strength you prefer.

SCALLOPS ROMA

Servings: 1 Lunch Entrée (4 blocks)

Block Size:	Ingredients:
4 Protein	6 ounces bay scallops
1 Carbohydrate	3 cups mushrooms, sliced
1½ Carbohydrate	1½ cups asparagus, cuts and tips
½ Carbohydrate	½ cup onion, chopped
1 Carbohydrate	½ cup Zoned Italian Sauce (see page 150)
4 Fat	1⅓ teaspoons olive oil, divided

Spices:

½ teaspoon dried dill
⅛ teaspoon lemon herb seasoning
⅛ teaspoon celery salt
⅛ teaspoon dried oregano
Pepper to taste

Method:

Heat ⅔ teaspoon oil in a medium nonstick sauté pan. Sauté scallops until cooked through. Stir in Zoned Italian Sauce and simmer 3 to 5 minutes. In second nonstick sauté pan, heat remaining oil and add mushrooms, asparagus, onion, dill, lemon herb seasoning, pepper, celery salt, and oregano. Cook until crisp-tender, about 5 minutes. Place vegetables on serving plate and top with scallop mixture.

SPICED PEPPER STEAK

Servings: 1 Lunch Entrée (4 blocks)

Block Size:	Ingredients:
4 Protein	4 ounces lean beef, thinly sliced
1 Carbohydrate	3 cups mushrooms, sliced
1 Carbohydrate	½ cup Zoned Herb Dressing (see page 156)
1 Carbohydrate	2¼ cups red and green pepper strips
1 Carbohydrate	1 cup onion, sliced
4 Fat	1⅓ teaspoons olive oil

Spices:

⅛ teaspoon Worcestershire sauce
2 tablespoons cider vinegar
⅛ teaspoon garlic powder

Method:

Heat oil in medium nonstick sauté pan. Sprinkle garlic powder onto beef. Sauté beef until cooked. Deglaze pan with Worcestershire sauce and vinegar. Add vegetables and stir-fry 5 to 7 minutes. Combine beef and vegetables in medium bowl and add Zoned Herb Dressing. Toss to coat. Spoon onto plate and serve.

BEEF AND VEGETABLE CASSEROLE

Servings: 1 Lunch Entrée (4 blocks)

Block Size:

4 Protein	4 ounces lean beef, diced
½ Carbohydrate	1½ cups cabbage, shredded (or coleslaw mix)
½ Carbohydrate	1½ cups mushrooms, sliced
½ Carbohydrate	¼ cup carrots, sliced
½ Carbohydrate	2 teaspoons cornstarch
1 Carbohydrate	1½ cups tomato, chopped
1 Carbohydrate	1 cup onion, chopped
4 Fat	1⅓ teaspoons olive oil

Spices:

2 tablespoons balsamic vinegar
½ teaspoon garlic, minced
⅛ teaspoon celery salt
¼ teaspoon dried cilantro
1 tablespoon Worcestershire sauce
3 tablespoons lime-flavored water

Method:
In a large nonstick sauté pan, lightly sauté beef in hot oil until just browned. Deglaze the pan with vinegar, Worcestershire sauce, and water. Combine all ingredients (except tomato, cornstarch, and cilantro) in pan and cook until tender. Stir in tomatoes and cornstarch and cook, stirring, for 3 to 5 minutes, until tomatoes are heated through and liquid thickens. (Mix cornstarch with a little water to dissolve it before adding to pan.) Spoon onto serving casserole. Sprinkle with cilantro and serve.

ITALIAN-STYLE PORK CUTLET

Servings: 1 Lunch Entrée (4 blocks)

Block Size:	Ingredients:
3 Protein	3 ounces pork cutlet
1 Protein	1 ounce skim milk mozzarella, shredded
1 Carbohydrate	½ cup Zoned Italian Sauce (see page 150)
½ Carbohydrate	1½ cups mushrooms, sliced
1 Carbohydrate	1 cup onion, chopped
1 Carbohydrate	1 cup Italian-style green beans
½ Carbohydrate	½ cup broccoli florets
4 Fat	1⅓ teaspoons olive oil, divided

Spices:

1 tablespoon dry red wine
¼ teaspoon dried oregano
½ teaspoon Worcestershire sauce
⅛ teaspoon dried rosemary
1 tablespoon lemon-flavored water
½ teaspoon garlic, minced
Dash ground thyme
Salt and pepper to taste

Method:
Place cutlet between two pieces of plastic wrap. Pound with a meat mallet until ⅛-inch thick. Heat 1 teaspoon oil in nonstick sauté pan over medium-high heat. Place cutlet in pan and sauté until done. Add Zoned Italian Sauce and simmer 3 to 5 minutes. In second nonstick sauté pan heat remaining oil. Sauté mushrooms, onion, beans, broccoli, wine, oregano, Worcestershire sauce, rosemary, thyme, water, garlic, and salt and pepper. Simmer mixture for 3 to 5 minutes. Spoon vegetables onto serving plate, top with cutlet, sprinkle with cheese, and serve.

TEX-MEX BEEF STIR-FRY

Servings: 1 Lunch Entrée (4 blocks)

Block Size:	Ingredients:
3 Protein	3 ounces lean beef, diced
1 Protein	1 ounce taco cheese, shredded
1 Carbohydrate	1¼ cup tomatoes, chopped
1 Carbohydrate	½ cup salsa*
1 Carbohydrate	¼ cup black beans, rinsed
1 Carbohydrate	2¼ cups red bell pepper strips
4 Fat	1⅓ teaspoons olive oil

Spices:

1 teaspoon chili powder or to taste
½ teaspoon garlic, minced
⅛ teaspoon ground cumin
¼ teaspoon ground red pepper (or
⅛ teaspoon hot pepper sauce)
1 tablespoon lemon-flavored water

Method:

In nonstick sauté pan heat oil over medium-high heat. Add beef and stir-fry 2 to 3 minutes. Stir in tomatoes, salsa, black beans, peppers, chili powder, garlic, cumin, red pepper, and water. Simmer until vegetables are tender, about 3 to 5 minutes. Spoon into serving bowl and top with cheese.

*Note: Salsa comes with different levels of heat. Choose one that best fits your family's tastes.

BARBECUE TURKEY TIPS WITH SPINACH SALAD

Servings: 1 Lunch Entrée (4 blocks)

Block Size:	Ingredients:
4 Protein	4 ounces turkey breast, 1-inch cubes
1 Carbohydrate	½ cup Zoned Barbecue Sauce (see page 154)
1 Carbohydrate	½ cup salsa*
½ Carbohydrate	½ cup onion, chopped
1 Carbohydrate	¼ cup chickpeas, rinsed and chopped
½ Carbohydrate	3 cups fresh spinach
4 Fat	1⅓ teaspoons olive oil

Method:

In a medium nonstick sauté pan, heat oil. Add turkey and sauté until cooked through. Blend in Zoned Barbecue Sauce, salsa, and onion. Simmer for 3 to 5 minutes. Arrange spinach on serving plate. Sprinkle spinach with chickpeas. Top spinach with turkey mixture and serve.

*Note: We used medium-heat salsa. Use whatever strength you prefer.

NATIVE AMERICAN CHICKEN WITH VEGETABLES

Servings: 1 Lunch Entrée (4 blocks)

Block Size:	Ingredients:
4 Protein	4 ounces chicken tenderloins, diced
1 Carbohydrate	¼ cup frozen corn kernels
½ Carbohydrate	½ cup onion, diced
1 Carbohydrate	¼ cup cooked black beans, rinsed
½ Carbohydrate	1½ cups mushrooms, sliced
1 Carbohydrate	1 cup whole green beans
4 Fat	1⅓ teaspoons olive oil, divided

Spices:

¼ teaspoon lemon herb seasoning
½ teaspoon Worcestershire sauce
⅛ teaspoon celery seed
½ teaspoon garlic, minced
Salt and pepper to taste

Method:

In a medium nonstick sauté pan, heat ⅔ teaspoon oil. Add chicken and lemon herb seasoning. Sauté until cooked through. In second nonstick sauté pan, heat remaining oil and sauté the corn, onion, black beans, mushrooms, green beans, Worcestershire sauce, celery seed, garlic, and salt and pepper. Cook until vegetables are crisp-tender. Blend chicken with vegetables and serve.

TACO BURGER

Servings: 1 Lunch Entrée (4 blocks)

Block Size:	Ingredients:
1 Protein	1 ounce low-fat jack cheese, shredded
3 Protein	4½ ounces lean (90 percent fat free) ground beef
1 Carbohydrate	1 taco shell, in pieces
1 Carbohydrate	½ cup salsa, divided*
½ Carbohydrate	2 cups lettuce, shredded
1 Carbohydrate	¼ cup cooked black beans, rinsed
½ Carbohydrate	½ cup onion, chopped
4 Fat	1⅓ teaspoons olive oil, divided

Spices:

½ teaspoon garlic, minced
½ teaspoon Worcestershire sauce
⅛ teaspoon celery salt
1 tablespoon lemon- or lime-flavored spring water

Method:

In a small bowl, combine ground beef and ¼ cup salsa. Form into a patty. Heat ⅔ teaspoon oil in a medium nonstick sauté pan and sauté patty until cooked through. In a second nonstick sauté pan, heat remaining oil. Place beans, garlic, ¼ cup salsa, onion, Worcestershire sauce, celery salt, and water in second sauté pan. Cook until heated through. Layer lettuce onto plate. Add patty, sprinkle with taco pieces, and top with bean mixture and cheese.

*Note: We used medium-heat salsa. Use whatever strength you prefer.

PORK AND VEGETABLE POCKET SANDWICH

Servings: 1 Lunch Entrée (4 blocks)

Block Size:	Ingredients:
3 Protein	3 ounces pork cutlet, finely sliced
1 Protein	1 ounce low-fat cheddar cheese, shredded
1 Carbohydrate	½ mini pita pocket
¼ Carbohydrate	¼ cup onion, chopped
¼ Carbohydrate	¼ cup asparagus pieces
¼ Carbohydrate	¾ cup bean sprouts
¼ Carbohydrate	½ tomato, sliced
½ Carbohydrate	¼ cup blueberries
½ Carbohydrate	½ cup raspberries
1 Carbohydrate	¾ cup cantaloupe cubes
1 Fat	1 teaspoon almonds, sliced
3 Fat	1 teaspoon olive oil

Spices:

½ teaspoon garlic, minced
1 teaspoon soy sauce
Dash celery salt
Dash lemon herb seasoning

Method:

Heat oil in medium nonstick sauté pan. Stir-fry pork until lightly browned. Add onion, asparagus, sprouts, garlic, soy sauce, celery salt, and lemon herb seasoning. Cook until asparagus is tender. Stir cheese into pork and blend it in as it melts. Place tomato slices in pita pocket. Spoon in pork mixture and place on serving plate. In a dessert bowl combine melon, berries, and almonds.

ORANGE HERBED CHICKEN STEW

Servings: 1 Lunch Entrée (4 blocks)

Block Size:	Ingredients:
4 Protein	4 ounces chicken tenderloin, diced
1 Carbohydrate	⅓ cup orange juice
2 Carbohydrate	⅔ cup Mandarin orange slices
1 Carbohydrate	3 cups mushrooms, sliced
4 Fat	1⅓ teaspoons olive oil, divided

Spices:

1 tablespoon cider vinegar
1 tablespoon parsley, chopped
½ teaspoon garlic, chopped
½ teaspoon pure orange extract
Salt and pepper to taste

Method:

In a medium nonstick sauté pan, heat ⅔ teaspoon oil. Add chicken, vinegar, parsley, garlic, and salt and pepper. In a second nonstick sauté pan heat remaining oil and sauté mushrooms until they soften. Add orange juice, orange slices, and orange extract to the first pan and simmer for 3 minutes. Place mushrooms in a serving bowl and top with chicken mixture.

MARYLAND-STYLE SEAFOOD CHOWDER

Servings: 1 Lunch Entrée (4 blocks)

Block Size:	Ingredients:
1½ Protein	2¼ ounces medium shrimp, large dice*
1½ Protein	2¼ ounces scallops, large dice
1 Protein and 1 Carbohydrate	1 cup 1 percent milk
½ Carbohydrate	½ cup onions, diced
½ Carbohydrate	1 cup celery, diced
½ Carbohydrate	¼ cup water chestnuts, diced
1 Carbohydrate	1¼ cups tomato, chopped
½ Carbohydrate	2 teaspoons cornstarch
4 Fat	1⅓ teaspoons olive oil

Spices:

1 teaspoon garlic, minced
1 cup chicken stock
1 tablespoon parsley
1 tablespoon cilantro
½ teaspoon Worcestershire sauce
Dash hot pepper sauce

Method:
In a medium nonstick sauté pan add oil, onions, water chestnuts, celery, parsley, cilantro, Worcestershire sauce, and hot pepper sauce. Cook until onion and celery are tender, then add shrimp, scallops, and garlic. Cook an additional 3 to 5 minutes, until shrimp are pink and scallops are opaque. Transfer to medium saucepan. Stir in tomato and chicken stock. Bring to a boil, reduce heat, cover and simmer for 7 minutes. Add milk and continue to simmer for 3 minutes. Dissolve

cornstarch in a little of the stock from the pot. Pour into saucepan and continue cooking, stirring frequently, until stock thickens.

Note: Shelled and deveined.

GRILLED SHRIMP SALAD

Servings: 1 Lunch Entrée (4 blocks)

Block Size:	Ingredients:
4 Protein	6 ounces raw shrimp*
½ Carbohydrate	1½ cups green cabbage, shredded
½ Carbohydrate	1½ cups red cabbage, shredded
1 Carbohydrate	1¼ cups chopped tomatoes
½ Carbohydrate	1¼ cups red pepper strips
½ Carbohydrate	1 cup green pepper strips
1 Carbohydrate	¼ cup chickpeas, rinsed
4 Fat	1⅓ teaspoons olive oil, divided

Spices:

½ teaspoon paprika
¼ teaspoon ground coriander
1 teaspoon garlic, minced, divided
1 tablespoon cider vinegar
1 tablespoon fresh parsley
1 tablespoon fresh basil, chopped
Dash cayenne pepper
Salt and pepper to taste

Method:
In a medium nonstick sauté pan add ⅓ teaspoon oil, paprika, coriander, cayenne, parsley, basil, and ½ teaspoon garlic. Heat spices on medium-high heat for 1 minute, then stir in shrimp and coat with seasonings. Stir-fry shrimp in spices until shrimp are pink. In a salad bowl combine

cabbage, tomatoes, peppers, and chickpeas. In small bowl whisk 1 teaspoon oil, vinegar, and remaining garlic. Pour over vegetables and gently toss to coat. Arrange on serving plate and top with shrimp.

Note: Shelled and deveined.

HAWAIIAN-STYLE FILLET OF SOLE SALAD

Servings: 1 Lunch Entrée (4 blocks)

Block Size:	Ingredients:
4 Protein	6 ounce fillet of sole
½ Carbohydrate	3 cups lettuce, shredded
½ Carbohydrate	1½ cups bean sprouts
1 Carbohydrate	2¼ cups red and green pepper strips
½ Carbohydrate	¼ cup carrots, shredded
1½ Carbohydrate	¾ cup pineapple, diced
4 Fat	1⅓ teaspoons olive oil, divided

Spices:

4 teaspoons soy sauce
2 teaspoons garlic, minced, divided
1 tablespoon cilantro
⅛ teaspoon lemon herb seasoning
2 tablespoons scallions, finely diced (for garnish)
2 tablespoons hot chili peppers, finely diced (for garnish)

Method:

In a small nonstick sauté pan, heat ⅓ teaspoon oil. Add 1 teaspoon garlic and cook for 1 minute. Sauté sole in same pan, 2 to 3 minutes per side, until it flakes easily. In salad bowl combine lettuce, sprouts, peppers, carrots, and pineapple. In a small bowl whisk together remaining oil, garlic, and soy sauce. Pour over vegetables and toss to coat. Flake sole and add to salad. Sprinkle with chopped lemon herb seasoning, scallions, chili peppers, and cilantro.

GARDEN SALAD TOPPED WITH SAUTÉED SCALLOPS AND BACON

Servings: 1 Lunch Entrée (4 blocks)

Block Size:	Ingredients:
1 Protein	1 ounce Canadian bacon, diced
3 Protein	4½ ounces bay scallops
½ Carbohydrate	3 cups lettuce, shredded
1 Carbohydrate	⅓ cup mandarin oranges
½ Carbohydrate	½ cup red onion, diced
1 Carbohydrate	¼ cup kidney beans, rinsed
1 Carbohydrate	¼ cup chickpeas, rinsed
4 Fat	1⅓ teaspoons olive oil, divided

Spices:

1 tablespoon cider vinegar, divided
½ teaspoon fresh mint, chopped
½ teaspoon fresh gingerroot, grated, divided
¼ cup chicken stock

Method:
Heat ⅓ teaspoon oil in medium nonstick sauté pan. Sauté bacon, scallops, 1 teaspoon vinegar, and ¼ teaspoon ginger for 4 minutes on medium-high heat. In a small bowl whisk together remaining oil, mint, ¼ teaspoon ginger, 2 teaspoons vinegar, and chicken stock. Combine remaining ingredients in a salad bowl. Add bacon and scallops. Pour in dressing and toss to coat.

CHINESE SEAFOOD SALAD

Servings: 1 Lunch Entrée (4 blocks)

Block Size:	Ingredients:
1 Protein	1½ ounces small cooked shrimp*
1 Protein	1½ ounces cooked bay scallops
1 Protein	1½ ounces canned salmon, flaked
1 Protein and 1 Carbohydrate	½ cup plain low-fat yogurt
½ Carbohydrate	½ cup scallions, thinly sliced
½ Carbohydrate	3 cups lettuce, shredded
½ Carbohydrate	½ cup tomatoes, diced
½ Carbohydrate	½ cucumber, grated
½ Carbohydrate	1 cup red and green pepper strips
¼ Carbohydrate	½ cup radishes, grated
¼ Carbohydrate	¼ cup snow peas, diced
4 Fat	4 teaspoons light mayonnaise

Spices:

⅛ teaspoon cayenne pepper
1 tablespoon cilantro
⅛ teaspoon dill
Lemon herb seasoning
Dash hot pepper sauce

Method:

In a medium bowl blend shrimp, scallops, salmon, scallions, light mayonnaise, dill, and hot pepper sauce. In second bowl mix together the yogurt, radishes, cucumber, cayenne, and cilantro. Combine yogurt dressing with lettuce, tomatoes, peppers, and snow peas. Top with seafood mixture, sprinkle with lemon herb seasoning, and serve.

*Note: Shelled and deveined.

SMOKED MACKEREL WITH RADISH AND ENDIVE

Servings: 1 Lunch Entrée (4 blocks)

Block Size:	Ingredients:
4 Protein	6 ounces smoked mackerel
½ Carbohydrate	1¼ cup radishes, sliced
½ Carbohydrate	1 cup red and green pepper strips
1 Carbohydrate	½ cup Zoned Herb Dressing (see page 156)
½ Carbohydrate	½ cup red onions, diced
1 Carbohydrate	½ Granny Smith apple, diced
½ Carbohydrate	3½ cups Belgian endive, chopped
4 Fat	1⅓ teaspoons olive oil

Spices:

2 teaspoons cider vinegar
Horseradish, grated (bottled or fresh to taste)
⅛ teaspoon dill
⅛ teaspoon dry mustard
Salt and pepper to taste

Method:

Combine mackerel, radishes, peppers, onion, apple, and endive in a medium salad bowl. In a blender combine oil, vinegar, horseradish, Zoned Herb Dressing, herbs, and salt and pepper. Pulse until well mixed. Pour over salad and toss gently to coat.

CURRIED TURKEY WITH LENTIL SALAD

Servings: 1 Lunch Entrée (4 blocks)

Block Size:	Ingredients:
3 Protein	4½ ounces deli-style turkey breast, finely chopped
1 Protein and 1 Carbohydrate	½ cup plain low-fat yogurt
1 Carbohydrate	¼ cup lentils, cooked
½ Carbohydrate	1 cup celery, chopped
½ Carbohydrate	½ cup red onion, sliced thinly
¼ Carbohydrate	1½ cups lettuce
¼ Carbohydrate	1½ cups romaine lettuce
¼ Carbohydrate	¾ cup bean sprouts
¼ Carbohydrate	1¼ cups escarole
4 Fat	6 teaspoons slivered almonds

Spices:

⅛ teaspoon curry
⅛ teaspoon cumin
⅛ teaspoon turmeric
⅛ teaspoon coriander
⅛ teaspoon cayenne pepper

Method:

In a medium bowl, combine turkey, yogurt, lentils, and spices. In a salad bowl, combine celery, onion, lettuce, romaine, sprouts, and escarole. Pour on yogurt mixture. Toss to coat and sprinkle with almonds.

GRILLED TURKEY SALAD WITH MANDARIN ORANGES

Servings: 1 Lunch Entrée (4 blocks)

Block Size:	Ingredients:
4 Protein	4 ounces turkey breast
½ Carbohydrate	1 cup celery, finely sliced
½ Carbohydrate	½ cup red onion, finely sliced
¼ Carbohydrate	1½ cups lettuce
¼ Carbohydrate	1½ cups romaine lettuce
1 Carbohydrate	½ cup Zoned French Dressing (see page 157)
1 Carbohydrate	⅓ cup Mandarin oranges
½ Carbohydrate	½ peach, diced
4 Fat	1⅓ teaspoons olive oil, divided

Spices:

⅛ teaspoon turmeric
1 tablespoon fresh mint, chopped

Method:
Heat ⅓ teaspoon oil in a small sauté pan. Add turkey and stir-fry until cooked through. In a salad bowl, combine turkey, celery, onion, 1 teaspoon oil, Zoned French Dressing, peach, oranges, turmeric, and mint. Toss lightly to coat. On a lunch plate place lettuce, and top with turkey mixture and serve.

MEDITERRANEAN CHICKEN SALAD WITH ARTICHOKE HEARTS

Servings: 1 Lunch Entrée (4 blocks)

Block Size:	Ingredients:
4 Protein	4 ounces chicken tenderloin, coarsely chopped
1 Carbohydrate	3 small artichoke hearts, chopped*
½ Carbohydrate	½ cup asparagus, 1-inch pieces
¼ Carbohydrate	¼ cup onion, chopped
½ Carbohydrate	1 cup red pepper, chopped
¼ Carbohydrate	½ cup celery, sliced
½ Carbohydrate	½ cup tomatoes, chopped
½ Carbohydrate	¼ cup chickpeas
¼ Carbohydrate	¾ cup lettuce, torn
¼ Carbohydrate	¾ cup romaine lettuce, torn
4 Fat	1⅓ teaspoons olive oil, divided

Spices:

1 tablespoon capers, chopped
1 teaspoon garlic, minced
1 tablespoon balsamic vinegar
1 tablespoon fresh basil, chopped
1 tablespoon fresh parsley, chopped
⅛ teaspoon chili powder
Salt and pepper to taste

Method:

In a medium nonstick sauté pan, sauté chicken in ⅓ teaspoon oil. Place remaining oil, capers, garlic, vinegar, and herbs and spices in a small bowl. Whisk to blend. In medium bowl combine artichokes, asparagus, onion, pepper, celery, and chicken. In a salad bowl combine the lettuce, romaine, chickpeas, and tomato. Pour dressing over salad and toss gently to coat. Top with chicken mixture and serve.

Note: 3 small artichoke hearts equal 1 medium artichoke.

STIR-FRY CHICKEN AND SNOW PEAS

Servings: 1 Lunch Entrée (4 blocks)

Block Size:	Ingredients:
4 Protein	4 ounces chicken tenderloin
½ Carbohydrate	3 cups spinach
1 Carbohydrate	¼ cup white kidney beans
½ Carbohydrate	1½ cups mushrooms, sliced
1 Carbohydrate	1 cup snow peas
½ Carbohydrate	1½ cups bean sprouts
½ Carbohydrate	½ cup scallions, sliced
4 Fat	1⅓ teaspoons olive oil

Spices:

½ cup chicken stock
2 teaspoons soy sauce
1 teaspoon cider vinegar
2 teaspoons Chinese five-spice powder
Hot pepper sauce to taste

Method:
Using a nonstick sauté pan, stir-fry chicken in hot chicken stock for 2 minutes. Add mushrooms and cook 3 minutes. Stir in kidney beans, snow peas, sprouts, and scallions. Cook 2 minutes more. In a small bowl mix oil, soy sauce, vinegar, five-spice powder, and hot sauce. Whisk to blend. In a salad bowl combine spinach, chicken, and vegetables (use slotted spoon to remove from sauté pan.) Pour dressing over salad and toss to coat.

GRILLED PORK WITH LENTIL SALAD

Servings: 1 Lunch Entrée (4 blocks)

Block Size:	Ingredients:
3½ Protein	3½ ounces lean pork
½ Protein and	
½ Carbohydrate	¼ cup plain low-fat yogurt
1 Carbohydrate	¼ cup lentils, cooked
½ Carbohydrate	½ cup carrot, shredded
¼ Carbohydrate	½ cup celery, sliced
¼ Carbohydrate	¼ cup red onion, sliced thinly
1 Carbohydrate	⅓ cup Mandarin orange sections
¼ Carbohydrate	1 cup romaine lettuce
¼ Carbohydrate	1¼ cups escarole
4 Fat	1⅓ teaspoons olive oil, divided

Spices:

1 teaspoon garlic, minced, divided
½ teaspoon dried oregano
⅛ teaspoon curry powder
1 tablespoon cilantro
½ teaspoon Worcestershire sauce
¼ teaspoon cumin
1 tablespoon cider vinegar
Salt and pepper to taste

Method:

In a medium nonstick sauté pan, heat 1 teaspoon oil. Blend in the curry powder, orange sections, vinegar, ½ teaspoon garlic, oregano, and salt and pepper. Add pork and cook until pork is cooked through. In a small bowl mix yogurt, remaining oil, garlic, cilantro, Worcestershire sauce, and cumin. Place the lettuce, escarole, onion, lentils, carrot, and celery in a salad bowl. Add yogurt mixture and toss to coat. Place salad mixture on a serving plate, top with pork mixture, and serve.

TOMATO BASIL SALAD

Servings: 1 Lunch Entrée (4 blocks)

Block Size:	Ingredients:
4 Protein	4 ounces skim milk mozzarella cheese, shredded
1 Carbohydrate	1¼ cups tomatoes, sliced
1 Carbohydrate	¼ cup chickpeas, rinsed and finely chopped
1 Carbohydrate	4 cups romaine lettuce, chopped
½ Carbohydrate	¼ cup Zoned Herb Dressing (see page 156)
½ Carbohydrate	¼ cup salsa*
4 Fat	1⅓ teaspoons olive oil

Spices:

1 tablespoon red wine vinegar
2 tablespoons fresh basil, chopped
1 tablespoon fresh parsley, chopped
1 teaspoon garlic, minced
¼ teaspoon chili powder

Method:

In a medium bowl combine lettuce, salsa, and Zoned Herb Dressing, then form into a bed on a serving plate. In a second bowl, blend chickpeas, parsley, oil, vinegar, basil, garlic, and chili powder. Alternate slices of tomato and shredded mozzarella on lettuce bed. Pour chickpea dressing over tomatoes and serve.

*Note: We used a medium-heat salsa. Use whatever strength you prefer.

GINGER-GARLIC STIR-FRY

Servings: 1 Lunch Entrée (4 blocks)

Block Size:	Ingredients:
4 Protein	12 ounces extra-firm tofu, ½-inch cubes
1 Carbohydrate	2 cups broccoli florets
½ Carbohydrate	½ cup asparagus spears
½ Carbohydrate	½ cup red onion, thinly sliced
½ Carbohydrate	½ cup scallions, sliced
½ Carbohydrate	1 cup celery, sliced
1 Carbohydrate	⅓ cup water chestnuts, sliced
4 Fat	1⅓ teaspoons olive oil, divided

Spices:

2 teaspoons garlic, minced (or to taste)
1 tablespoon cider vinegar
½ teaspoon Chinese five-spice powder
½ teaspoon Worcestershire sauce
⅛ teaspoon celery salt
2 teaspoons fresh gingerroot, minced
1 tablespoon soy sauce
Salt and pepper to taste

Method:

Heat ⅔ teaspoon oil in medium nonstick sauté pan. When hot, add Worcestershire sauce, celery salt, and tofu. Stir-fry until tofu is browned and crusted on all sides. In second nonstick sauté pan heat remaining oil. Add in broccoli, asparagus, onion, celery, scallions, water chestnuts, garlic, vinegar, five-spice powder, gingerroot, soy sauce, and salt and pepper. Stir-fry until vegetables are crisp-tender, about 5 minutes. Place vegetables on serving plate and top with tofu.

SAUTÉED GREEN BEANS WITH TOFU

Servings: 1 Lunch Entrée (4 blocks)

Block Size:	Ingredients:
4 Protein	12 ounces extra-firm tofu, 1-inch cubes
3 Carbohydrate	3 cups green beans, 2-inch pieces
1 Carbohydrate	1 cup onion, chopped
4 Fat	1⅓ teaspoons olive oil, divided

Spices:

½ teaspoon garlic, minced
½ teaspoon Worcestershire sauce
⅛ teaspoon celery salt
2 teaspoons cider vinegar
⅛ teaspoon nutmeg
⅛ teaspoon cinnamon
⅛ teaspoon lemon herb seasoning
⅛ teaspoon ground double superfine mustard
½ teaspoon soy sauce
Salt and pepper to taste

Method:

Heat ⅔ teaspoon oil in medium nonstick sauté pan. Blend in Worcestershire sauce, celery salt, and tofu. Stir-fry tofu until browned and crusted on all sides. In a second nonstick sauté pan, heat remaining oil and add in green beans, onion, garlic, vinegar, nutmeg, cinnamon, lemon herb seasoning, mustard, soy sauce, and salt and pepper. Cook until beans are crisp-tender. Place beans on serving plate and top with tofu.

MUSTARD-GLAZED BRUSSELS SPROUTS WITH TOFU

Servings: 1 Lunch Entrée (4 blocks)

Block Size:	Ingredients:
4 Protein	12 ounces extra-firm tofu, ½-inch dice
2 Carbohydrate	3 cups brussels sprouts, frozen
1 Carbohydrate	1 cup red onion, chopped
1 Carbohydrate	½ cup Zoned Tarragon Mustard Sauce (see page 160)
4 Fat	1⅓ teaspoons olive oil, divided

Spices:

1 teaspoon garlic, minced
½ teaspoon Worcestershire sauce
⅛ teaspoon celery salt
Salt and pepper to taste

Method:

Heat ⅔ teaspoon oil in a medium nonstick sauté pan. Blend in Worcestershire sauce, celery salt, and tofu. Stir-fry until browned and crusted on all sides. In a medium saucepan cook brussels sprouts according to package directions. Remove from pan and drain. In a second nonstick sauté pan, heat remaining oil and garlic. Stir in sprouts, Zoned Tarragon Mustard Sauce, and onion. Stir-fry until onion is tender. Place sprout mixture on serving plate and top with tofu.

CITRUS TOFU SALAD

Servings: 1 Lunch Entrée (4 blocks)

Block Size:	Ingredients:
4 Protein	12 ounces extra-firm tofu, ½-inch dice
1 Carbohydrate	1 cup asparagus spears, 1-inch pieces
½ Carbohydrate	1 cup celery, sliced
½ Carbohydrate	1½ cups romaine lettuce
2 Carbohydrate	⅔ cup Mandarin orange segments
4 Fat	1⅓ teaspoons olive oil, divided

Spices:

½ teaspoon garlic, minced
Dash hot pepper sauce
½ teaspoon paprika
⅛ teaspoon lemon herb seasoning
½ teaspoon Worcestershire sauce
⅛ teaspoon celery salt
½ teaspoon dried dill
Salt and pepper to taste

Method:

In a medium nonstick sauté pan, heat ⅔ teaspoon oil. Blend in Worcestershire sauce, celery salt, and tofu. Stir-fry until browned and crusted on all sides. In a second nonstick sauté pan, heat remaining oil and stir-fry the asparagus, celery, garlic, hot pepper sauce, paprika, lemon herb seasoning, dill, and salt and pepper until vegetables are crisp-tender. Place lettuce on serving plate. Distribute orange segments over lettuce. Top first with vegetable mixture, then with tofu.

CANADIAN-STYLE SPINACH SALAD

Servings: 1 Lunch Entrée (4 blocks)

Block Size:	Ingredients:
4 Protein	4 ounces Canadian bacon, diced
½ Carbohydrate	3 cups spinach*
1 Carbohydrate	1 cup canned mushrooms, sliced
½ Carbohydrate	½ cup scallions, sliced (white and green parts)
1 Carbohydrate	½ cup Zoned Herb Dressing (see page 156)
1 Carbohydrate	½ Granny Smith apple, cored and chopped
4 Fat	1⅓ teaspoons olive oil, divided

Spices:

2 teaspoons balsamic vinegar
½ teaspoon Dijon mustard
Salt and pepper to taste

Method:

In a nonstick sauté pan, heat ⅓ teaspoon oil. Lightly brown the Canadian bacon in the oil. Blend 1 teaspoon oil, balsamic vinegar, mustard, and salt and pepper into the Zoned Herb Dressing. Combine spinach, mushrooms, scallions, apple, and bacon in serving bowl. Add dressing, toss to coat, and serve.

*Note: Fresh spinach needs to be cleaned very well, because of its tendency to have sand in it, so be sure to soak spinach in water to remove any sand or dirt before using.

GRILLED SOLE WITH LEEKS

Servings: 1 Lunch Entrée (4 blocks)

Block Size:	Ingredients:
4 Protein	6 ounces fillet of sole
3 Carbohydrate	3 cups leeks, sliced
1 Carbohydrate	4 ounces Johannesburg Riesling
4 Fat	1⅓ teaspoons olive oil, divided

Spices:

1 teaspoon garlic, minced
1 shallot, minced*
½ teaspoon lemon herb seasoning
1 teaspoon dill
Salt and pepper to taste

Method:
Brush a medium baking dish with oil. Layer bottom of dish with leeks. Place sole on top. In a medium bowl combine wine, garlic, shallot, dill, and salt and pepper. Gently pour wine mixture into baking dish. Sprinkle with lemon herb seasoning. Tightly cover baking dish and place in a preheated 375 degrees Fahrenheit oven. Bake for 25 to 30 minutes and serve.

Note: Shallots are available in most supermarkets and have a purple-white appearance. Shallots provide dishes with both an onion and garlic flavor.

FRUIT SALAD WITH PEPPER RELISH

Servings: 1 Lunch Entrée (4 blocks)

Block Size:

4 Protein

1 Carbohydrate

1 Carbohydrate
½ Carbohydrate
½ Carbohydrate
1 Carbohydrate

4 Fat

Ingredients:

1 cup low-fat cottage cheese

½ Granny Smith apple, cored and chopped

⅓ cup mandarin orange sections
2 cups romaine
1½ teaspoons raisins
¾ cup Zoned Pepper Relish (see page 159)

4 macadamia nuts, chopped

Spices:

Salt and pepper to taste

Method:
Form a bed of romaine on a serving plate. Top with Zoned Pepper Relish. In a medium bowl, combine cheese, apple, orange sections, raisins, and salt and pepper. Mix well. Mound cheese on top of lettuce and sprinkle with nuts.

GINGER TURKEY WITH ORIENTAL VEGETABLES

Servings: 1 Lunch Entrée (4 blocks)

Block Size:	Ingredients:
3 Protein	4½ ounces lean ground turkey
1 Protein	2 egg whites
1 Carbohydrate	⅓ cup water chestnuts, finely chopped
½ Carbohydrate	½ cup scallions, finely chopped, divided
1 Carbohydrate	1 cup canned mushrooms, minced, divided
½ Carbohydrate	1½ cups cabbage, shredded
½ Carbohydrate	1½ cups bean sprouts
½ Carbohydrate	1 cup celery, sliced
4 Fat	1⅓ teaspoons olive oil, divided

Spices:

¼ teaspoon curry powder
½ teaspoon chili powder
½ teaspoon garlic, minced
2 tablespoons lemon- and lime-flavored water
2 teaspoons cilantro, chopped
4 teaspoons soy sauce
Salt and pepper to taste

Method:

In a small bowl combine turkey, egg white, 1 teaspoon soy sauce, ¼ cup mushrooms, ¼ cup scallions, water chestnuts, and salt and pepper. Mix well and form into a patty. Heat ⅓ teaspoon oil in a small nonstick sauté pan. Sauté patty until cooked through. In a medium-sized nonstick sauté pan heat remaining oil. Add ¼ cup scallions, ¾ cup mushrooms, cabbage, bean sprouts, celery, curry powder, chili powder, garlic, cilantro, 3 teaspoons soy sauce, lemon- and lime-water, and salt and pepper. Cook until crisp-tender. Spoon vegetables onto serving plate and top with patty.

ITALIAN-STYLE CHICKEN

Servings: 1 Lunch Entrée (4 blocks)

Block Size:	Ingredients:
4 Protein	4 ounces chicken tenderloin, sliced diagonally
1 Carbohydrate	1 cup onion, chopped
1 Carbohydrate	¼ cup chickpeas, rinsed
1 Carbohydrate	1¼ cups plum tomatoes, chopped
1 Carbohydrate	6 cups spinach, chopped
4 Fat	1⅓ teaspoons olive oil, divided

Spices:

½ cup chicken stock
½ teaspoon Worcestershire sauce
1 teaspoon garlic, chopped
1½ teaspoon dried oregano
Salt and pepper to taste

Method:
In a medium nonstick sauté pan, heat ⅔ teaspoon oil. Add chicken, ½ cup onion and Worcestershire sauce. In a second nonstick sauté pan heat remaining oil. Stir in ½ cup onion, chickpeas, plum tomatoes, spinach, stock, garlic, oregano, and salt and pepper. Sauté until spinach begins to wilt. Place vegetable mixture on serving plate and top with chicken.

STIR-FRY CHICKEN WITH GINGER VEGETABLES

Servings: 1 Lunch Entrée (4 blocks)

Block Size:	Ingredients:
4 Protein	4 ounces chicken tenderloin, ½-inch cubes
½ Carbohydrate	1½ cups mushrooms, sliced
1 Carbohydrate	1½ cups cabbage, shredded
½ Carbohydrate	½ cup snow peas
1 Carbohydrate	⅓ cup water chestnuts
½ Carbohydrate	½ cup scallion, ¼-inch pieces
½ Carbohydrate	½ cup cauliflower florets
4 Fat	1⅓ teaspoons olive oil, divided

Spices:

1 tablespoon soy sauce
¼ cup chicken broth
2 teaspoons fresh gingerroot, minced, divided
1 teaspoon garlic, minced, divided

Method:

Heat ⅔ teaspoon oil in a medium nonstick sauté pan. Add chicken, ½ teaspoon ginger, and ½ teaspoon garlic. Stir-fry until chicken is cooked and garlic is lightly browned. In a second nonstick sauté pan heat remaining oil and stir in mushrooms. Cook for 2 minutes. Add cabbage, snow peas, water chestnuts, scallions, cauliflower, soy sauce, broth, and remaining ginger and garlic. Stir-fry until cabbage and cauliflower are tender. Place vegetables on serving dish and top with chicken.

BAKED CHICKEN AND ITALIAN VEGETABLE PACKAGES

Servings: 1 Lunch Entrée (4 blocks)

Block Size:	Ingredients:
4 Protein	4 ounces chicken tenderloin, finely diced
1 Carbohydrate	1 cup zucchini, ⅛-inch slices
1 Carbohydrate	1 cup onion, thinly sliced
1 Carbohydrate	⅓ cup red potato, thinly sliced
1 Carbohydrate	1¼ cup tomato, seeded and chopped
4 Fat	1⅓ teaspoons olive oil

Spices:

1 tablespoon balsamic vinegar
2 teaspoons garlic, minced
1 teaspoon dried thyme
1 teaspoon dried oregano
4 tablespoons parsley, chopped
Salt and pepper to taste

Method:

Preheat oven to 425 degrees Fahrenheit. Combine chicken and vegetables in a medium bowl. In a small bowl whisk together olive oil, vinegar, garlic, thyme, oregano, parsley, and salt and pepper. Pour over chicken-vegetable mixture. Toss to coat. Cut a piece of aluminum foil large enough to wrap mixture. Place foil on baking tray and fill with mixture. Fold foil up around the mixture and seal it. Leave a small steam vent on the top of the package. Bake for 25 to 30 minutes. When done, cut open foil (be careful of escaping steam) and spoon mixture onto serving dish.

THAI TURKEY SOUP

Servings: 1 Lunch Entrée (4 blocks)

Block Size:	Ingredients:
4 Protein	6 ounces ground turkey
½ Carbohydrate	1½ cups bean sprouts
½ Carbohydrate	½ cup scallions, sliced
½ Carbohydrate	2 cups spinach leaves
1 Carbohydrate	¼ cup cooked fine egg noodles
1½ Carbohydrate	¾ cup fruit cocktail
4 Fat	1⅓ teaspoons olive oil

Spices:

3 teaspoons garlic, minced
½ teaspoon fresh gingerroot, grated
2 tablespoons soy sauce
2½ cups chicken stock
1 tablespoon hot chili pepper, finely diced

Method:
Combine turkey, sprouts, scallions, oil, garlic, gingerroot, soy sauce, stock, and chili pepper in a medium saucepan. Bring to a boil, reduce heat, and simmer for 15 minutes. Add spinach and noodles. Simmer for 1 minute. Spoon into serving bowl and serve with fruit cocktail as a side dish, in a second serving bowl.

VEGETABLE STEW

Servings: 1 Lunch Entrée (4 blocks)

Block Size:	Ingredients:
4 Protein	4 soy hot dogs, sliced
½ Carbohydrate	1 cup celery, sliced
1 Carbohydrate	1 cup scallions, sliced
1 Carbohydrate	½ cup carrots, finely diced
1 Carbohydrate	1¼ cups tomato, chopped
½ Carbohydrate	1½ cups mushrooms, sliced
4 Fat	1⅓ teaspoons olive oil

Spices:

2 teaspoons garlic, minced
3 cups beef stock
2 tablespoons cider vinegar
⅛ teaspoon Worcestershire sauce
⅛ teaspoon dried oregano
Salt and pepper to taste

Method:
Combine all ingredients in a large saucepan. Bring to a boil, then simmer for 35 to 40 minutes, stirring occasionally until all vegetables are tender. Place mixture in serving dish, and serve immediately.

DINNER

CHICKEN CREOLE

Servings: 1 Dinner Entrée (4 blocks)

Block Size:	Ingredients:
4 Protein	4 ounces chicken tenderloins, ½-inch cubes
1 Carbohydrate	1 cup onions, chopped
1 Carbohydrate	½ cup Zoned Italian Sauce (see page 150)
½ Carbohydrate	1½ cups mushrooms, sliced
½ Carbohydrate	1¼ cups celery, sliced
1 Carbohydrate	2¼ cups red and green pepper strips
4 Fat	1⅓ teaspoons olive oil

Spices:

1 teaspoon chili powder
½ teaspoon dry red wine
1 teaspoon garlic, minced
Hot pepper sauce to taste (optional)

Method:

Heat oil in medium nonstick sauté pan. Add chicken, onion, mushrooms, celery, pepper strips, chili powder, wine, and garlic. Stir-fry until chicken is cooked and vegetables are tender. Stir in Zoned Italian Sauce and cook an additional 3 minutes. Spoon onto plate and serve.

MUSHROOM SAUCE STEAK WITH MIXED VEGETABLES

Servings: 1 Dinner Entrée (4 blocks)

Block Size:	Ingredients:
4 Protein	4 ounces lean beef, thinly sliced
1 Carbohydrate	1 cup Zoned Mushroom Sauce (see page 148)
1 Carbohydrate	1 cup asparagus pieces
½ Carbohydrate	½ cup onion, chopped
½ Carbohydrate	1 cup cauliflower florets
1 Carbohydrate	1 cup whole green beans
4 Fat	1⅓ teaspoons olive oil

Spices:

1 teaspoon garlic, minced
½ teaspoon Worcestershire sauce

Method:
Sauté beef and garlic in hot oil until cooked. Add Zoned Mushroom Sauce and Worcestershire sauce. Simmer for 3 minutes, until heated through. Steam vegetables until crisp-tender (4 to 5 minutes). Place vegetables on one side of serving plate and spoon saucy beef onto the other.

SHEPHERD'S PIE

Servings: 1 Dinner Entrée (4 blocks)

Block Size:	Ingredients:
3 Protein	4½ ounces lean ground beef
1 Protein	¼ cup egg substitute
½ Carbohydrate	¼ cup tomato puree
½ Carbohydrate	1½ cups mushrooms, sliced
1 Carbohydrate	¼ cup frozen corn kernels
1 Carbohydrate	1 cup turnip, diced
½ Carbohydrate	½ cup green beans
½ Carbohydrate	½ cup onion, chopped
4 Fat	1⅓ teaspoons olive oil, divided

Spices:

2 tablespoons beef stock, divided
1 teaspoon Worcestershire sauce
⅛ teaspoon celery seed
⅛ teaspoon dried marjoram
1 tablespoon balsamic vinegar
⅛ teaspoon lemon herb seasoning
1 cup water
Salt and pepper to taste

Method:
In a medium nonstick sauté pan heat ⅓ teaspoon of oil. Add ground beef, egg substitute, ½ teaspoon Worcestershire sauce, and celery seed. Stir-fry until cooked. Blend in tomato puree and marjoram. Cook an additional 3 minutes. In a second nonstick sauté pan heat 1 teaspoon oil, mushrooms, corn, green beans, onion, vinegar, ½ teaspoon Worcestershire sauce, 1 tablespoon beef stock, lemon herb seasoning, and salt and pepper. While the beef mixture and mushroom mixture are cooking, place diced turnip and 1 cup of water in a saucepan and

cook until turnip softens. Drain water from saucepan and mash turnip. Layer a small casserole dish with beef mixture. Sprinkle with 1 tablespoon beef stock. Add mushroom mixture on top of beef mixture and place a layer of turnip on mushroom mixture. Brown casserole in broiler and serve.

Note: This recipe is simple to prepare and reheats well in a microwave or toaster oven.

OLD-FASHIONED ITALIAN PIE

Servings: 1 Dinner Entrée (4 blocks)

Block Size:	Ingredients:
1 Protein	¼ cup egg substitute
1 Protein	2 ounces skim milk ricotta cheese (approximately ¼ cup)
2 Protein	3 ounces lean ground beef
1 Carbohydrate	½ cup Zoned Italian Sauce (see page 150)
½ Carbohydrate	¼ cup tomato puree
½ Carbohydrate	½ cup onion, chopped
1 Carbohydrate	1½ cups broccoli florets
1 Carbohydrate	1 cup frozen asparagus pieces
4 Fat	1⅓ teaspoons olive oil, divided

Spices:

½ teaspoon garlic, minced
⅛ teaspoon dried marjoram
⅛ teaspoon dried oregano
Dash ground nutmeg
¼ teaspoon lemon herb seasoning
½ teaspoon Worcestershire sauce
Salt and pepper to taste

Method:

In a medium nonstick sauté pan heat ⅔ teaspoon of oil, beef, cheese, egg substitute, Worcestershire sauce, garlic, marjoram, oregano, nutmeg, salt and pepper until beef is cooked. In a second nonstick sauté pan heat ⅔ teaspoon oil and sauté the onion, broccoli, asparagus, and lemon herb seasoning. Cook until vegetables are crisp-tender. Add Zoned Italian-Style Sauce and tomato puree. Simmer 3 to 5 minutes. In a small casserole dish alternate layers of meat and vegetables. Place in microwave and heat through.

GERMAN BEEF SALAD

Servings: 1 Dinner Entrée (4 blocks)

Block Size:	Ingredients:
4 Protein	4 ounces cooked lean beef, thinly sliced
1 Carbohydrate	1 cup onion, thinly sliced
½ Carbohydrate	3 cups fresh spinach
½ Carbohydrate	1 cup celery, sliced
1 Carbohydrate	1 cup sauerkraut, drained
1 Carbohydrate	½ cup Zoned Herb Dressing (see page 156)
4 Fat	1⅓ teaspoons olive oil

Spices:

½ teaspoon Worcestershire sauce

Method:

In small nonstick sauté pan heat oil. Add beef and brown. Stir in Zoned Herb Dressing and Worcestershire sauce. Remove from heat. On serving plate, layer spinach, sauerkraut, celery, and onion. Top with meat mixture and serve.

SPICED BEANS WITH MUSHROOMS

Servings: 1 Dinner Entrée (4 blocks)

Block Size:	Ingredients:
4 Protein	12 ounces extra-firm tofu, ½-inch cubes
½ Carbohydrate	½ cup green beans
1 Carbohydrate	3 cups mushrooms, sliced
½ Carbohydrate	½ cup onions, chopped
1 Carbohydrate	½ cup Zoned Herb Dressing
1 Carbohydrate	¼ cup cooked black beans, rinsed
4 Fat	1⅓ teaspoons olive oil, divided

Spices:

⅛ teaspoon celery salt
½ teaspoon Worcestershire sauce
1 tablespoon balsamic vinegar
¼ teaspoon lemon and herb seasoning

Method:

Heat ⅔ teaspoon oil in a medium nonstick sauté pan. Sauté tofu, celery salt, and Worcestershire sauce until well browned and crusted on all sides. In a second nonstick sauté pan, heat remaining oil. Add green beans, mushrooms, onions, black beans, balsamic vinegar, and lemon and herb seasoning. Sauté until vegetables are crisp-tender, about 3 to 5 minutes. Mix tofu with vegetables. Add Zoned Herb Dressing, heat through, and serve.

SWEET AND SOUR SHRIMP SALAD

Servings: 1 Dinner Entrée (4 blocks)

Block Size:	Ingredients:
4 Protein	6 ounces cooked shrimp
1 Carbohydrate	½ cup canned pineapple, cubed
1 Carbohydrate	1 cup snow peas, 1-inch pieces
½ Carbohydrate	½ cup onion, chopped
½ Carbohydrate	¾ cup canned bean sprouts
1 Carbohydrate	½ cup Zoned Barbecue Sauce (see page 154)
4 Fat	1⅓ teaspoons olive oil

Spices:

½ teaspoon garlic, minced
2 tablespoons lemon-flavored water

Method:
Heat oil in a medium nonstick sauté pan. Add snow peas, onion, and sprouts. Sauté until crisp-tender. Stir in pineapple, water, Zoned Barbecue Sauce, and garlic. Cook an additional 3 to 5 minutes. Add shrimp and heat through. Spoon into a medium bowl and serve.

SHRIMP GUMBO

Servings: 1 Dinner Entrée (4 blocks)

Block Size:	Ingredients:
4 Protein	6 ounces small shrimp*
½ Carbohydrate	1 cup celery, sliced
1 Carbohydrate	1 cup onion, chopped
1 Carbohydrate	1¼ cups tomatoes, chopped
½ Carbohydrate	½ cup frozen okra, sliced
1 Carbohydrate	¼ cup frozen corn kernels
4 Fat	1⅓ teaspoons olive oil

Spices:

½ teaspoon hot pepper sauce
  (or to taste)
½ teaspoon garlic, minced
¼ teaspoon chili powder
⅛ teaspoon celery seed
⅓ cup lemon- and lime-flavored
  water
½ teaspoon lemon herb
  seasoning
¼ teaspoon paprika

Method:

Heat oil in a medium nonstick sauté pan. Add celery, onion, tomatoes, okra, corn, hot pepper sauce, garlic, chili powder, and celery seed. Cook until vegetables are tender. Mix in the shrimp, paprika, lemon herb seasoning, and water. Simmer 3 to 5 minutes until the shrimp are cooked. Spoon into a medium bowl and serve.

*Note: Shelled and deveined.

WARMED DILL TUNA SALAD

Servings: 1 Dinner Entrée (4 blocks)

Block Size:	Ingredients:
4 Protein	4 ounces albacore tuna, canned in water
½ Carbohydrate	5½ cups alfalfa sprouts
1 Carbohydrate	½ cup salsa*
½ Carbohydrate	½ cup tomato, chopped
½ Carbohydrate	3 cups lettuce, shredded
½ Carbohydrate	½ cup onion, chopped, divided
1 Carbohydrate	½ cup Zoned Herb Dressing (see page 156)
4 Fat	1⅓ teaspoons olive oil

Spices:

1 teaspoon dill

Method:

Heat oil in a medium nonstick sauté pan. In a medium bowl combine tuna, sprouts, salsa, and dill. Add to sauté pan. Sauté until heated through and lightly browned. On a serving plate, form the lettuce into a bed and top with tomato and onion. Spoon on tuna mixture and sprinkle with Zoned Herb Dressing.

*Note: We used a medium-heat salsa. Use whatever strength you prefer.

STIR-FRY SALMON WITH SNOW PEAS

Servings: 1 Dinner Entrée (4 blocks)

Block Size:	Ingredients:
3 Protein	4½ ounces canned salmon
1 Protein	1 whole egg
½ Carbohydrate	½ cup onion, chopped
1 Carbohydrate	1 cup fresh snow peas
1 Carbohydrate	⅓ cup water chestnuts, sliced
1 Carbohydrate	½ cup salsa*
½ Carbohydrate	1½ cups mushrooms, sliced
4 Fat	1⅓ teaspoons olive oil, divided

Spices:

1 teaspoon dill
1 teaspoon Worcestershire sauce
1 tablespoon balsamic vinegar
⅛ teaspoon celery seed
⅛ teaspoon dry ground double
   superfine mustard

Method:

Heat ⅔ teaspoon oil in a medium nonstick sauté pan. Combine salmon, egg, salsa, and dill. Sauté until heated through. Heat remaining oil in a second pan. Add onion, snow peas, water chestnuts, mushrooms, Worcestershire sauce, vinegar, celery seed, and mustard. Sauté until vegetables are tender. Combine salmon mixture with vegetables and serve.

Note: We used a medium-heat salsa. Use whatever strength you prefer.

GOURMET GARDENBURGERS

Servings: 1 Dinner Entrée (4 blocks)

Block Size:	Ingredients:
4 Protein	6 ounces lean ground beef
1 Carbohydrate	1 cup Zoned Mushroom Sauce (see page 148)
1 Carbohydrate	3 cups bean sprouts, divided
½ Carbohydrate	2 cups cucumber, peeled, seeded, and chopped
1 Carbohydrate	¼ cup kidney beans, rinsed
½ Carbohydrate	½ cup onion, chopped
4 Fat	1⅓ teaspoons olive oil, divided

Spices:

1 teaspoon Worcestershire sauce
½ teaspoon garlic, minced
⅛ teaspoon dried oregano
⅛ teaspoon celery seed
Dash chili powder
⅛ teaspoon lemon herb seasoning
Salt and pepper to taste

Method:

Heat ⅔ teaspoon olive oil in a medium nonstick sauté pan. In a medium bowl combine the beef, 1½ cups sprouts, Worcestershire sauce, garlic, celery seed, oregano, and chili powder. Form into four small patties. Sauté patties in hot oil until cooked. Add in Zoned Mushroom Sauce and heat through. In a second nonstick sauté pan, heat remaining oil. Add 1½ cups sprouts, cucumber, kidney beans, onion, and lemon herb seasoning. Sauté until the vegetables start to soften. Drain excess liquid from vegetables. Spoon into a small serving bowl. Place burgers onto a serving dish with more Zoned Mushroom Sauce.

STIR-FRY PORK WITH TARRAGON-MUSTARD SAUCE

Servings: 1 Dinner Entrée (4 blocks)

Block Size:	Ingredients:
4 Protein	4 ounces pork strips, thinly sliced
1 Carbohydrate	½ cup Zoned Tarragon Mustard Sauce (see page 160)
1 Carbohydrate	1 cup onion, chopped
1 Carbohydrate	¼ cup kidney beans, rinsed
1 Carbohydrate	2¼ cups frozen red and green bell pepper strips
4 Fat	1⅓ teaspoons olive oil, divided

Spices:

2 teaspoons Worcestershire sauce
1 tablespoon lemon-flavored water

Method:

Heat ⅔ teaspoon oil in a medium sauté pan. Add pork and water to pan and stir-fry until meat is cooked. Spoon in Zoned Tarragon Mustard Sauce and heat through. In second nonstick sauté pan, heat remaining oil. Place onion, beans, peppers, and Worcestershire sauce in second pan and stir-fry until tender. Place vegetables on a serving plate. Top with meat mixture and serve.

PORK CUTLET TUSCAN-STYLE

Servings: 1 Dinner Entrée (4 blocks)

Block Size:	Ingredients:
4 Protein	4 ounces pork cutlets
1 Carbohydrate	1 cup onion, chopped
½ Carbohydrate	¼ cup tomato puree
1 Carbohydrate	½ cup Zoned Herb Dressing, divided (see page 156)
1 Carbohydrate	¼ cup canned chickpeas, chopped
½ Carbohydrate	1½ cups mushrooms, sliced
4 Fat	1⅓ teaspoons olive oil, divided

Spices:

½ teaspoon ground double superfine mustard

⅛ teaspoon black pepper

1 teaspoon Worcestershire sauce

2 tablespoons lemon- or lime-flavored water

Method:

Blend mustard, pepper, Worcestershire sauce, and ¼ cup Zoned Herb Dressing in a small bowl. Heat ⅔ teaspoon oil in a nonstick sauté pan. Add mustard mixture and water to pan. Place cutlets and onion in pan. Make sure to coat both sides of cutlets with mustard mixture. In a second nonstick pan heat remaining oil. Add chickpeas and mushrooms. Cook for 3 to 5 minutes. Stir in tomato puree and ¼ cup Zoned Herb Dressing. Simmer for an additional 2 minutes. Combine vegetables and pork. Blend well and spoon onto a serving plate.

SOUTH AMERICAN CHILI SOUP

Servings: 1 Dinner Entrée (4 blocks)

Block Size:	Ingredients:
4 Protein	4 ounces chicken tenderloin, chopped
1 Carbohydrate	2¼ cups frozen red and green pepper strips
1 Carbohydrate	½ cup salsa*
1 Carbohydrate	1¼ cups tomatoes, chopped
½ Carbohydrate	½ cup onion, chopped
½ Carbohydrate	2 teaspoons cornstarch
4 Fat	1⅓ teaspoons olive oil

Spices:

1 teaspoon Worcestershire sauce
1 tablespoon balsamic vinegar
⅛ teaspoon hot pepper sauce
1 cup chicken stock
½ teaspoon garlic, minced
¼ teaspoon chili powder

Method:

In a nonstick sauté pan heat oil. Sauté chicken, onion, peppers, salsa, Worcestershire sauce, vinegar, and hot pepper sauce until lightly browned. In large saucepan combine chicken mixture, tomatoes, chicken stock, garlic, chili powder, and cornstarch. (Mix cornstarch with chicken stock before adding to saucepan.) Bring mixture to a simmer, stirring constantly, for 3 to 5 minutes. Spoon into bowl and serve.

*Note: We used medium-heat salsa. Use whatever strength you prefer.

DEVILED STEAK WITH MIXED VEGETABLES

Servings: 1 Dinner Entrée (4 blocks)

Block Size:	Ingredients:
4 Protein	4 ounces lean beef
1 Carbohydrate	3 cups mushrooms, sliced
1 Carbohydrate	¼ cup frozen corn kernels
1 Carbohydrate	1 cup asparagus cuts
½ Carbohydrate	½ cup onion, chopped
½ Carbohydrate	¼ cup tomato puree
4 Fat	1⅓ teaspoons olive oil

Spices:

½ teaspoon Worcestershire sauce
1 tablespoon balsamic vinegar
Dash ground cloves
1 teaspoon ground double superfine mustard
2 tablespoons lemon- and lime-flavored water
⅛ teaspoon celery salt

Method:

In a medium nonstick sauté pan, combine oil, Worcestershire sauce, vinegar, cloves, mustard, and water. Stir to mix well. Add meat to pan and sprinkle the meat with the celery salt. Cook 3 to 5 minutes. Add mushrooms, corn, asparagus, and onion. Sauté until vegetables are tender. Add tomato puree and simmer 3 to 5 minutes. Spoon onto plate and serve.

SWISS-STYLE CHICKEN

Servings: 1 Dinner Entrée (4 blocks)

Block Size:	Ingredients:
2 Protein	2 ounces chicken tenderloin, diced
1 Protein	1 ounce low-fat Swiss cheese, shredded
1 Protein and 1 Carbohydrate	½ cup plain low-fat yogurt
½ Carbohydrate	½ cup onion, chopped
½ Carbohydrate	3 cups spinach
1 Carbohydrate	1¼ cups tomato, diced
1 Carbohydrate	⅓ cup Mandarin orange slices
4 Fat	1⅓ teaspoons olive oil, divided

Spices:

Dash celery salt
2 tablespoons lemon- and lime-flavored water
½ teaspoon Worcestershire sauce
1 teaspoon parsley flakes
1 teaspoon garlic, minced
1 tablespoon cider vinegar
Dash ground nutmeg

Method:

In a medium nonstick sauté pan combine ⅓ teaspoon oil, yogurt, and celery salt. Add chicken, onion, Worcestershire sauce, parsley, and water. Simmer for 3 to 5 minutes. In second pan heat remaining oil. Add spinach, tomato, garlic, vinegar, and nutmeg. Sauté until spinach has wilted and tomato softened slightly. Sprinkle cheese over chicken and let melt. Spoon spinach onto serving plate and top with chicken. Garnish with orange segments and serve.

PORK TENDERLOIN WITH APPLE COMPOTE

Servings: 1 Dinner Entrée (4 blocks)

Block Size:	Ingredients:
4 Protein	4 ounces pork tenderloin
2 Carbohydrate	1 Granny Smith apple, cored and chopped
1 Carbohydrate	⅓ cup unsweetened applesauce
1 Carbohydrate	3 cups mushrooms, sliced
4 Fat	1⅓ teaspoons olive oil, divided
	2 tablespoons cider vinegar
	⅛ teaspoon celery salt
	⅛ teaspoon cinnamon
	2 tablespoons lemon- and lime-flavored water
	¼ teaspoon lemon herb seasoning

Method:

Heat ⅔ teaspoon of oil in a medium nonstick sauté pan. Sauté pork loin until cooked through and lightly browned. Add apple, applesauce, vinegar, celery salt, cinnamon, water, and lemon herb seasoning. Simmer for 3 to 5 minutes. In second nonstick sauté pan, heat remaining oil. Add mushrooms and cook for 3 to 5 minutes. Spoon mushrooms onto a serving plate. Top with pork mixture and serve.

HUNGARIAN CHICKEN

Servings: 1 Dinner Entrée (4 blocks)

Block Size:	Ingredients:
4 Protein	4 ounces chicken tenderloin, cut in large chunks
1 Carbohydrate	1¼ cups tomatoes, chopped
1 Carbohydrate	2¼ cups green and red pepper strips
1 Carbohydrate	1 cup onion, chopped
1 Carbohydrate	¼ cup chickpeas, rinsed
4 Fat	1⅓ teaspoons olive oil, divided

Spices:

Dash hot red pepper sauce (optional)
1 tablespoon paprika
1 teaspoon Worcestershire sauce
½ teaspoon garlic, minced
⅛ teaspoon celery seed
Salt and pepper to taste

Method:

Heat ⅔ teaspoon oil in a medium nonstick sauté pan. Add chicken, sprinkle with salt and pepper. Cook chicken until lightly browned. In a second nonstick sauté pan, heat remaining oil and cook tomatoes, pepper strips, onion, chickpeas, hot pepper sauce, paprika, Worcestershire sauce, garlic, and celery seed. Sauté vegetables and seasonings for 3 to 5 minutes, until they begin to soften. Spoon vegetables onto a serving dish and top with chicken.

CHICKEN MEXICALI SALAD

Servings: 1 Dinner Entrée (4 blocks)

Block Size:	Ingredients:
3 Protein	3 ounces chicken tenderloin, large dice
1 Protein and 1 Carbohydrate	½ cup plain low-fat yogurt
1 Carbohydrate	½ cup salsa*
½ Carbohydrate	1½ cups cabbage, shredded (¾ cup red cabbage and ¾ cup green cabbage)
½ Carbohydrate	¼ cup Zoned Herb Dressing (see page 156)
1 Carbohydrate	3 cups mushrooms, sliced
4 Fat	1⅓ teaspoons olive oil, divided

Spices:

1 tablespoon cider vinegar
⅛ teaspoon hot pepper sauce
Celery salt and black pepper
    to taste

Method:

In a medium nonstick sauté pan add ⅔ teaspoon oil, chicken, mushrooms, and salsa and cook 3 to 5 minutes stirring occasionally. Add vinegar, hot pepper sauce, and Zoned Herb Dressing to chicken mixture, stirring constantly, heating throughout. Remove from heat and stir in the yogurt and raw cabbage. Spoon onto serving plate and sprinkle lightly with celery salt and black pepper.

*Note: We used medium-heat salsa. Use whatever strength you prefer.

SUMMER VEGETABLES WITH GARLIC STIR-FRY

Servings: 1 Dinner Entrée (4 blocks)

Block Size:	Ingredients:
4 Protein	12 ounces extra-firm tofu, diced
1 Carbohydrate	1¼ cups tomato, chopped
½ Carbohydrate	1 cup celery, sliced
1 Carbohydrate	1½ cups zucchini, large dice
½ Carbohydrate	½ cup scallion, 1-inch pieces
1 Carbohydrate	½ cup Zoned Italian Sauce (see page 150)
4 Fat	1⅓ teaspoons olive oil, divided

Spices:

½ teaspoon parsley flakes
½ teaspoon Worcestershire sauce
⅛ teaspoon celery salt
⅛ teaspoon lemon herb seasoning
⅛ teaspoon dried oregano
1 tablespoon dry red wine
Dash ground thyme
1 tablespoon lemon-flavored water
1 tablespoon garlic, minced
Salt and pepper to taste

Method:

In a medium nonstick sauté pan heat ⅔ teaspoon oil. Add Worcestershire sauce and celery salt. Stir in tofu and stir-fry until tofu is browned and crusted on all sides. In a second nonstick sauté pan heat remaining oil and sauté tomato, celery, zucchini, scallion, Zoned Italian Sauce, parsley, lemon herb seasoning, oregano, wine, thyme, water, garlic, and salt and pepper. Cook vegetables until they are tender. Place browned tofu in bottom of serving bowl and spoon vegetables on top.

PEPPER STIR-FRY

Servings: 1 Dinner Entrée (4 blocks)

Block Size:	Ingredients:
4 Protein	12 ounces extra-firm tofu, diced
½ Carbohydrate	2 teaspoons cornstarch
1 Carbohydrate	1¼ cups tomatoes, chopped
1 Carbohydrate	2¼ cups red and yellow bell peppers, chopped
½ Carbohydrate	½ cup onion, chopped
1 Carbohydrate	¼ cup chickpeas, rinsed
4 Fat	1⅓ teaspoons olive oil, divided

Spices:

⅛ teaspoon celery salt
½ teaspoon Worcestershire sauce
1 teaspoon garlic, minced
1 tablespoon cider vinegar
Dash hot pepper sauce
⅛ teaspoon paprika
⅓ cup lemon- and lime-flavored water
Dash lemon herb seasoning

Method:
In a medium nonstick sauté pan, heat ⅔ teaspoon of oil. Add tofu, celery salt, and Worcestershire sauce and stir-fry until browned and crusted on all sides. In a second pan heat remaining oil. Add peppers, onion, chickpeas, garlic, vinegar, hot pepper sauce, and paprika. Cook until the vegetables are tender. Add tomatoes, water, and cornstarch. (Mix cornstarch with water to dissolve it before adding to sauté pan.) Combine tofu and vegetable mixture. Spoon onto serving plate and sprinkle with lemon herb seasoning.

COUNTRY-STYLE TURKEY WITH GREEN BEANS

Servings: 1 Dinner Entrée (4 blocks)

Block Size:	Ingredients:
4 Protein	6 ounces lean ground turkey
½ Carbohydrate	1 cup celery, finely diced, divided
1 Carbohydrate	1 cup green beans, 2-inch pieces
1 Carbohydrate	1¼ cups cherry tomatoes, halved
½ Carbohydrate	½ cup leeks, finely diced
1 Carbohydrate	1 cup Zoned Country-Style Chicken Gravy (see page 149)
4 Fat	1⅓ teaspoons olive oil, divided

Spices:

½ teaspoon Worcestershire sauce
½ teaspoon garlic, minced, divided
⅛ teaspoon parsley, minced
Dash black pepper
⅛ teaspoon chili powder

Method:

In a medium mixing bowl, combine turkey, ½ cup celery, leeks, Worcestershire sauce, and parsley. Form into ½-inch meatballs. Coat a baking dish with ⅔ teaspoon oil. Place meatballs in baking dish. Bake in a preheated 370-degree Fahrenheit oven for 15 minutes. In a medium nonstick sauté pan heat remaining oil. Add remaining celery, green beans, cherry tomatoes, garlic, black pepper, and chili powder. Cook until vegetables are tender. Stir in Zoned Country-Style Chicken Gravy. Heat through and serve.

CHICKEN ZUCCHINI ITALIANO

Servings: 1 Dinner Entrée (4 blocks)

Block Size:

1 Protein	1 ounce skim milk mozzarella, shredded
3 Protein	3 ounces chicken tenderloin, finely diced
2 Carbohydrate	3 cups zucchini, sliced
1 Carbohydrate	½ cup Zoned Italian Sauce (see page 150)
½ Carbohydrate	1½ cups mushrooms, diced
½ Carbohydrate	½ cup onion, chopped
4 Fat	1⅓ teaspoons olive oil

Spices:

1 tablespoon fresh basil, chopped
2 teaspoons garlic, minced
⅛ teaspoon dried oregano

Method:
In a medium nonstick sauté pan add oil, chicken, zucchini, mushrooms, onion, basil, garlic, and oregano. Sauté until vegetables are tender, then add Zoned Italian Sauce. Spoon into serving bowl and top with cheese.

POLYNESIAN-STYLE SHRIMP AND FRUIT STEW

Servings: 1 Dinner Entrée (4 blocks)

Block Size:	Ingredients:
4 Protein	6 ounces cooked shrimp
1 Carbohydrate	½ cup pineapple, cubed
½ Carbohydrate	2 teaspoons cornstarch
½ Carbohydrate	3 cups kale
1 Carbohydrate	½ cup honeydew melon, cubed
1 Carbohydrate	⅓ cup Mandarin orange segments
4 Fat	1⅓ teaspoons olive oil, divided

Spices:

½ cup lemon- and lime-flavored
  water
½ teaspoon lemon extract
½ teaspoon orange extract
¼ teaspoon Worcestershire sauce
1 teaspoon cider vinegar
Dash lemon herb seasoning

Method:

Heat ⅔ teaspoon oil in a medium nonstick sauté pan. Add kale and cook until just wilted. Remove to serving bowl. In a second pan heat remaining oil and stir in the shrimp, pineapple, melon, orange segments, water, lemon extract, orange extract, Worcestershire sauce, vinegar, and lemon herb seasoning. Sauté until orange breaks up. Mix cornstarch with a little water to dissolve it and add to sauté pan, stirring constantly, until liquid thickens slightly. On large lunch plate spoon shrimp fruit mixture over kale and serve.

PORTUGUESE-STYLE PORK WITH CLAMS

Servings: 1 Dinner Entrée (4 blocks)

Block Size:	Ingredients:
3 Protein	3 ounces pork loin, sliced ⅛-inch thick
1 Protein	1½ ounces clams
½ Carbohydrate	½ cup onions, sliced
1 Carbohydrate	¾ Zoned Pepper Relish
1 Carbohydrate	¼ cup chickpeas, diced
1 Carbohydrate	2 cups celery, sliced
½ Carbohydrate	½ cup white wine
4 Fat	1⅓ teaspoons olive oil

Spices:

2 teaspoons garlic
1 tablespoon parsley flakes
Dash hot pepper sauce
⅛ teaspoon paprika
2 teaspoons cider vinegar

Method:

In a glass bowl, combine the vinegar, oil, and garlic. Add pork and turn in liquid to coat. Cover and refrigerate for 30 minutes. When pork is marinated add pork and liquid to a medium nonstick sauté pan. Stir in remaining ingredients and sauté until pork is cooked through. Spoon onto dish and serve.

PORK MEDALLIONS WITH PEAR AND BLUEBERRY COMPOTE

Servings: 1 Dinner Entrée (4 blocks)

Block Size:	Ingredients:
4 Protein	4 ounces pork loin, sliced ⅛-inch thick
1½ Carbohydrate	1½ pears, diced
½ Carbohydrate	2 cups romaine lettuce, shredded
1 Carbohydrate	2 teaspoons brown sugar, divided
½ Carbohydrate	¼ cup blueberries
½ Carbohydrate	½ cup scallion, shredded
4 Fat	1⅓ teaspoons olive oil, divided

Spices:

½ teaspoon soy sauce
1 tablespoon lemon- and lime-flavored water
2 teaspoons mint, minced
2 teaspoons Dijon mustard
1 tablespoon cider vinegar
2 tablespoons red wine vinegar
⅛ teaspoon celery salt
⅛ teaspoon black pepper

Method:
In a glass bowl, combine ⅔ teaspoon oil, mustard, cider vinegar, and 1 teaspoon brown sugar. Add pork and turn to coat. Cover and refrigerate for 30 minutes. When pork is done marinating add the mixture to a medium nonstick sauté pan. Sauté until the pork is cooked through. Stir in the pears, blueberries, 1 teaspoon brown sugar, mint, and water. In a medium bowl mix together the ⅔ teaspoon oil, soy sauce, red wine vinegar, scallions, romaine, celery salt, and black pepper. Spoon vegetable mixture onto serving plate and top with pork and fruit mixture.

HOT AND SOUR STIR-FRY PORK AND CABBAGE

Servings: 1 Dinner Entrée (4 blocks)

Block Size:	Ingredients:
4 Protein	4 ounces lean pork loin, large dice
¼ Carbohydrate	1 teaspoon cornstarch
¼ Carbohydrate	½ cup cauliflower pieces
½ Carbohydrate	½ cup onion, sliced
½ Carbohydrate	½ cup scallions, chopped
½ Carbohydrate	1½ cups cabbage, shredded
2 Carbohydrate	1 pear, cored and sliced
4 Fat	1⅓ teaspoons olive oil

Spices:

½ cup chicken stock
1 tablespoon soy sauce
⅛ teaspoon black pepper
2 tablespoons jalapeño peppers, diced
1 tablespoon cider vinegar
2 teaspoons minced garlic
2 teaspoons fresh gingerroot, minced

Method:
In a medium glass bowl combine the oil, pork, stock, cornstarch, soy sauce, vinegar, scallions, and spices. Cover and refrigerate for 30 minutes. When the pork is done marinating, place mixture in a medium nonstick sauté pan. Sauté pork until browned on both sides, then add vegetables and continue cooking until vegetables are tender. Place pork and vegetables on a large dinner plate, garnished with pear slices. Serve immediately.

SPICED GROUND LAMB WITH SPRING VEGETABLES

Servings: 1 Dinner Entrée (4 blocks)

Block Size:	Ingredients:
4 Protein	6 ounces lean ground lamb
½ Carbohydrate	½ cup scallions, finely chopped
½ Carbohydrate	½ cup red onion, chunks
½ Carbohydrate	1½ cups mushrooms
1 Carbohydrate	1¼ cups tomatoes, diced
½ Carbohydrate	½ cup green beans, diced
1 Carbohydrate	⅕ cup cooked brown rice
4 Fat	1⅓ teaspoons olive oil

Spices:

1 teaspoon cider vinegar
1 tablespoon cilantro
2 teaspoons gingerroot, minced
¼ teaspoon cumin
¼ teaspoon coriander
⅛ teaspoon black pepper
½ teaspoon celery salt
⅛ teaspoon cinnamon

Method:

In a small glass bowl combine lamb, rice, vinegar, and spices. Cover and refrigerate for 30 minutes. Heat the oil in a medium nonstick sauté pan. Add meat mixture and vegetables. Cook, breaking meat up as it cooks, until lamb is cooked through and the vegetables are tender. Spoon onto plate and serve.

LAMB WITH SPICED BEANS

Servings: 1 Dinner Entrée (4 blocks)

Block Size:	Ingredients:
3 Protein	3 ounces lean lamb, finely diced
1 Protein and	
1 Carbohydrate	½ cup plain low-fat yogurt
½ Carbohydrate	½ cup onions, thinly sliced
1 Carbohydrate	3 cups cabbage, shredded
1 Carbohydrate	¼ cup cooked white kidney beans
½ Carbohydrate	3¾ cups escarole, chopped
4 Fat	1⅓ teaspoons olive oil

Spices:

2 teaspoons garlic, minced
½ teaspoon paprika
¼ teaspoon ground cumin
⅛ teaspoon cayenne pepper
⅛ teaspoon celery salt

Method:

In a glass bowl combine lamb, yogurt, paprika, cumin, garlic, cayenne, and celery salt. Mix well to coat. Cover and refrigerate for 4 hours. Heat oil in medium nonstick sauté pan. Add meat mixture and vegetables. Cook until lamb is cooked through and vegetables are tender.

BRAISED LAMB WITH KALE AND BEANS

Servings: 1 Dinner Entrée (4 blocks)

Block Size:	Ingredients:
4 Protein	4 ounces lean lamb, small dice
1 Carbohydrate	1 cup onions, sliced
1 Carbohydrate	1¼ cups kale, torn
1 Carbohydrate	½ Granny Smith apple, roughly chopped
1 Carbohydrate	¼ cup white kidney beans
4 Fat	1⅓ teaspoons olive oil

Spices:

½ cup lemon- and lime-flavored water
½ teaspoon ground cinnamon
⅛ teaspoon cayenne pepper
Salt and pepper to taste

Method:

In a small pan sauté lamb and onion in hot oil until lightly browned. Add water, cinnamon, cayenne, and salt and pepper. Cover, reduce heat, and simmer for 10 minutes. Add kale, apple, and beans. Bring to a boil, reduce heat, cover, and simmer for 2 minutes to heat through. Place lamb on serving dish, and using a slotted spoon, arrange vegetables on dish.

BRAISED BEEF WITH MIXED VEGETABLES

Servings: 1 Dinner Entrée (4 blocks)

Block Size:	Ingredients:
4 Protein	4 ounces lean beef, small dice
1 Carbohydrate	1 cup onion, roughly chopped
1 Carbohydrate	1 cup green beans, 2-inch pieces
½ Carbohydrate	1 cup celery, roughly chopped
½ Carbohydrate	1½ cups mushrooms, sliced
1 Carbohydrate	6 ounces beer (flat beer is acceptable)
4 Fat	1⅓ teaspoons olive oil

Spices:

¼ cup beef stock
⅛ teaspoon celery salt
⅛ teaspoon dried thyme
⅛ teaspoon Worcestershire sauce
⅛ teaspoon dried rosemary
1 teaspoon garlic, minced
⅛ teaspoon dried oregano
½ tablespoon fresh parsley, chopped

Method:

Combine ingredients in a medium saucepan. Bring to a boil, reduce heat and simmer, covered, 25 to 30 minutes. Place mixture in a large soup bowl and serve.

GRILLED STEAK WITH SPICED MUSHROOM SALAD

Servings: 1 Dinner Entrée (4 blocks)

Block Size:	Ingredients:
4 Protein	4 ounces lean beef
1 Carbohydrate	⅓ cup cooked potato, thinly sliced
½ Carbohydrate	½ cup red onion, thinly sliced
½ Carbohydrate	1½ cups mushrooms, thinly sliced
½ Carbohydrate	1 cup red pepper, thinly sliced
1 Carbohydrate	1 cup asparagus spears, chopped
½ Carbohydrate	½ cup scallions, chopped
4 Fat	1⅓ teaspoons olive oil, divided
	4 tablespoons balsamic vinegar, divided
	2 tablespoons Dijon mustard, divided
	½ teaspoon garlic, minced
	1 teaspoon Worcestershire sauce
	Salt and pepper to taste

Method:

In a medium bowl combine beef, ⅔ teaspoon oil, 2 tablespoons vinegar, mustard, and ½ teaspoon Worcestershire sauce. Turn meat to cover with mixture. Cover bowl and refrigerate for 4 hours. Heat remaining oil in a medium nonstick sauté pan. Sauté beef until cooked through. In a small bowl whisk together remaining vinegar, remaining Worcestershire sauce, garlic, salt and pepper. In another medium bowl combine the potato, onion, mushrooms, pepper, asparagus, and scallions. Pour on dressing and toss to coat. Spoon salad onto serving dish and top with meat.

HERB-MARINATED BEEF WITH SUMMER VEGETABLES

Servings: 1 Dinner Entrée (4 blocks)

Block Size:	Ingredients:
4 Protein	4 ounces lean beef, diced
1 Carbohydrate	2¼ cups red and green pepper strips
½ Carbohydrate	½ cup zucchini, chunks
½ Carbohydrate	½ cup yellow squash, chunks
½ Carbohydrate	1½ cups mushrooms, quartered
1 Carbohydrate	1¼ cups tomato, chopped
½ Carbohydrate	2 ounces dry red wine
4 Fat	1⅓ teaspoons olive oil, divided

Spices:

1 tablespoon balsamic vinegar
1 teaspoon Worcestershire sauce
1 teaspoon garlic, minced
1 tablespoon fresh basil, chopped
1 tablespoon fresh mint, chopped
1 tablespoon fresh parsley, chopped
Salt and pepper to taste

Method:
Combine ⅔ teaspoon oil with wine, vinegar, Worcestershire sauce, garlic, basil, mint, parsley, and salt and pepper. Add meat, turn to coat, cover, and refrigerate 4 hours. Heat remaining oil in medium nonstick sauté pan. Sauté beef, pepper, zucchini, squash, mushrooms, and tomatoes until beef is cooked through and vegetables are tender.

BEEF WITH PEACHES AND ROOT VEGETABLES

Servings: 1 Dinner Entrée (4 blocks)

Block Size:	Ingredients:
4 Protein	4 ounces lean beef, thinly sliced
1 Carbohydrate	1 cup onion, finely chopped
1 Carbohydrate	½ cup carrot, thinly sliced
1½ Carbohydrate	1½ peaches, large dice
½ Carbohydrate	1 cup celery, chopped
4 Fat	1⅓ teaspoons olive oil

Spices:

1 tablespoon red wine vinegar
1 tablespoon Dijon mustard
1 teaspoon garlic, minced
⅛ teaspoon celery salt
⅛ teaspoon dried thyme
⅛ teaspoon cayenne pepper

Method:

Heat oil in a medium nonstick sauté pan. Add beef, onion, carrot, peaches, celery, and seasonings. Stir-fry until beef is cooked through and vegetables are tender.

TOFU-EGGPLANT GUMBO

Servings: 1 Dinner Entrée (4 blocks)

Block Size:	Ingredients:
4 Protein	12 ounces extra-firm tofu, 1-inch cubes
½ Carbohydrate	½ cup onion, chopped
½ Carbohydrate	½ cup scallion, chopped
½ Carbohydrate	1¼ cups green pepper, chopped
½ Carbohydrate	¾ cup okra, sliced
½ Carbohydrate	1 cup celery, sliced
1 Carbohydrate	1¼ cups tomato, crushed
½ Carbohydrate	¾ cup eggplant, diced
4 Fat	1⅓ teaspoons olive oil, divided

Spices:

2 cups beef stock
2 teaspoons garlic, chopped
½ teaspoon dried thyme
⅛ teaspoon cayenne pepper
2 teaspoons Worcestershire sauce, divided
⅛ teaspoon celery salt
¼ cup fresh parsley, chopped

Method:

In a medium nonstick sauté pan heat ⅔ teaspoon oil. Stir in ½ teaspoon Worcestershire sauce and celery salt. Add tofu and stir-fry until browned and crusted on all sides. In a second nonstick sauté pan heat remaining oil. Place onion, scallion, green peppers, celery, tomato, and eggplant in pan. Sprinkle with remaining Worcestershire sauce and remaining spices. Cook vegetables until just tender. Add okra and beef stock. Continue cooking until liquid thickens. Spoon into serving bowl and top with tofu.

SPICY TOFU-VEGETABLE STIR-FRY

Servings: 1 Dinner Entrée (4 blocks)

Block Size:	Ingredients:
4 Protein	12 ounces extra-firm tofu
½ Carbohydrate	1½ cups mushrooms, sliced
¼ Carbohydrate	¼ cup onion, thinly sliced
1 Carbohydrate	1½ cups zucchini, sliced
½ Carbohydrate	1½ cups bean sprouts
½ Carbohydrate	2 teaspoons cornstarch
¼ Carbohydrate	½ cup red bell pepper, diced
¼ Carbohydrate	¼ cup scallions, 1-inch pieces
½ Carbohydrate	1 cup celery, chopped
¼ Carbohydrate	½ cup radishes, sliced
4 Fat	1⅓ teaspoons olive oil, divided

Spices:

⅛ teaspoon celery salt
½ teaspoon Worcestershire sauce
1 tablespoon soy sauce
1 teaspoon garlic, crushed
1 teaspoon gingerroot, grated
1 tablespoon cider vinegar
¼ teaspoon chili powder
1 cup lemon- and lime-flavored water

Method:

In a medium nonstick sauté pan heat ⅔ teaspoon oil. Stir in Worcestershire sauce and celery salt. Add tofu and stir-fry until browned and crusted on all sides. In another nonstick sauté pan cook vegetables in remaining oil until tender, then add ½ cup water and cover to steam sauté. In saucepan add ½ cup water, soy sauce, spices, and cornstarch. (Mix cornstarch with water to dissolve it before adding to saucepan.) Heat sauce to a light boil while constantly stirring, then add diced tofu to sauce and heat. Add tofu and sauce to vegetables, stir, and simmer for 2 to 3 minutes. On a large dinner plate place tofu-vegetable mixture and serve.

GINGER-GRILLED TUNA

Servings: 1 Dinner Entrée (4 blocks)

Block Size:	Ingredients:
4 Protein	4 ounces tuna steak
3 Carbohydrate	3 cups asparagus
1 Carbohydrate	½ cup Zoned Herb Dressing (see page 156)
4 Fat	1⅓ teaspoons olive oil, divided

Spices:

4 teaspoons cider vinegar
2 teaspoons soy sauce
1½ tablespoons scallions, sliced
1 tablespoon gingerroot, minced
1 teaspoon garlic, minced
Coarse ground black pepper to taste

Method:
In the bottom of a small baking dish place ⅔ teaspoon oil, then place tuna steak. In a small bowl combine remaining oil, vinegar, soy sauce, scallions, ginger, garlic, and pepper. Pour spice mixture over tuna. Cover and bake in a preheated 350-degree Fahrenheit oven for 30 to 35 minutes. Steam the asparagus until crisp-tender. Place asparagus on one side of a serving plate. Pour Zoned Herb Dressing over it. Remove tuna from baking dish and place on serving plate.

SWORDFISH WITH PEACH-CUCUMBER SALSA

Servings: 1 Dinner Entrée (4 blocks)

Block Size:	Ingredients:
4 Protein	4 ounces swordfish steak
1 Carbohydrate	1 peach, chopped
1 Carbohydrate	½ cup salsa*
½ Carbohydrate	2 cups cucumber, chopped
½ Carbohydrate	2 cups romaine
½ Carbohydrate	½ cup shallots, diced
½ Carbohydrate	¼ cup dry white wine
4 Fat	1⅓ teaspoons olive oil

Spices:

½ teaspoon dill
1 teaspoon lemon- and lime-
  flavored water
½ teaspoon lemon herb
  seasoning
Salt and pepper to taste

Method:
Place swordfish in a baking dish. Drizzle with water, oil, and wine. Sprinkle with dill, salt and pepper, and lemon herb seasoning. Cover and bake in a preheated 350-degree Fahrenheit oven for 30 to 35 minutes. In a small bowl combine chopped peaches, salsa, cucumber, and shallots. Place lettuce on one side of a large dinner plate. Spoon salsa mixture on top of lettuce, then place swordfish on the other side of plate and serve.

*Note: We used medium heat salsa. Use whatever strength you prefer.

CIOPPINO

Servings: 1 Dinner Entrée (4 blocks)

Block Size:	Ingredients:
1 Protein	1½ ounces cherrystone clams
1 Protein	1½ ounces sole
1 Protein	1½ ounces small shrimp*
1 Protein	1½ ounces baby bay scallops
½ Carbohydrate	½ cup onion, chopped
½ Carbohydrate	1 cup green pepper, chopped
1 Carbohydrate	1 cup canned tomato, chopped
1 Carbohydrate	3 cups mushrooms, chopped
1 Carbohydrate	4 ounces dry red wine
4 Fat	1⅓ teaspoons olive oil

Spices:

1 teaspoon garlic, minced
½ cup lemon- and lime-flavored water
1 tablespoon parsley, chopped (for garnish)
¼ teaspoon dried oregano
¼ teaspoon dried basil
⅛ teaspoon cayenne pepper
Salt and pepper to taste

Method:
In a medium saucepan combine oil, vegetables, spices, water, and wine. Bring to a boil, reduce heat and bring to a simmer. Add seafood, cover, and simmer for 5 to 7 minutes. Spoon into a bowl and serve.

*Note: Shelled and deveined.

INDIAN SHRIMP WITH APPLES AND YOGURT

Servings: 1 Dinner Entrée (4 blocks)

Block Size:	Ingredients:
3 Protein	
1 Protein and	
1 Carbohydrate	4½ ounces cooked small shrimp*
	½ cup plain low-fat yogurt
½ Carbohydrate	½ cup onion, minced
2 Carbohydrate	1 Granny Smith apple, diced
½ Carbohydrate	2 cups romaine
4 Fat	1⅓ teaspoons olive oil

Spices:

⅛ teaspoon fresh gingerroot, minced
½ teaspoon garlic, minced
1 tablespoon cilantro
2 teaspoons cider vinegar
Dash hot pepper sauce
¼ teaspoon turmeric
⅛ teaspoon ground coriander
⅛ teaspoon ground cumin

Method:
Heat the oil in a medium nonstick sauté pan. Add shrimp and spices. Cook 1 to 2 minutes. In a second nonstick sauté pan heat yogurt, apple, and onion. When heated through, add shrimp mixture. Stir to mix. Form a bed of romaine on a serving plate and top with shrimp mixture.

*Note: Shrimp should be deveined and shelled.

BAKED SALMON WITH FRUIT SALSA

Servings: 1 Dinner Entrée (4 blocks)

Block Size:	Ingredients:
4 Protein	6 ounces salmon steak
1 Carbohydrate	¾ cup blackberries
1 Carbohydrate	½ cup salsa*
1 Carbohydrate	1 kiwi fruit, peeled and diced
1 Carbohydrate	½ Granny Smith apple, diced
4 Fat	1⅓ teaspoons olive oil

Spices:

2 teaspoons soy sauce
1 teaspoon gingerroot, chopped
½ teaspoon dill
Dash hot pepper sauce

Method:
Brush baking dish with oil; place salmon steak in baking dish. Sprinkle with soy sauce, gingerroot, dill, and hot pepper sauce. Cover and bake in a preheated 350-degree Fahrenheit oven for 30 to 35 minutes. In a medium bowl combine salsa and fruit. Place fish on one side of a serving plate and salsa beside it.

*Note: We used a medium heat salsa. Use whatever strength you prefer.

SAUTÉD SCALLOPS WITH WINE-FLAVORED VEGETABLES

Servings: 1 Dinner Entrée (4 blocks)

Block Size:	Ingredients:
4 Protein	6 ounces baby bay scallops
½ Carbohydrate	¼ cup white wine
½ Carbohydrate	½ cup asparagus, chopped
2 Carbohydrate	6 small artichoke hearts, chopped*
½ Carbohydrate	1 cup red pepper, sliced
½ Carbohydrate	¼ cup Zoned French Dressing (see page 157)
4 Fat	1⅓ teaspoons olive oil, divided

Spices:

½ teaspoon garlic, minced
1 tablespoon fresh parsley, chopped
½ teaspoon Worcestershire sauce
Salt and pepper to taste

Method:

In a medium nonstick sauté pan heat ⅔ teaspoon oil. Add scallops, garlic, parsley, and Worcestershire sauce. Sauté until scallops are cooked through. In a second nonstick sauté pan add remaining oil, asparagus, artichokes, red pepper, and Zoned French Dressing. Cook until vegetables are crisp-tender. Add scallops and wine. Sauté an additional 3 to 5 minutes and spoon onto a serving dish. Salt and pepper to taste.

*Note: 3 small artichoke hearts equal 1 medium artichoke.

SAUTÉED TURKEY WITH APPLE-CHILI PEPPER RELISH

Servings: 1 Dinner Entrée (4 blocks)

Block Size:	Ingredients:
4 Protein	4 ounces turkey breast, diced (boneless, skinless)
1 Carbohydrate	1 cup red onion, chopped
1 Carbohydrate	¾ cup Zoned Pepper Relish (see page 159)
2 Carbohydrate	1 Granny Smith apple, chopped
4 Fat	1⅓ teaspoons olive oil

Spices:

1 tablespoon cider vinegar
½ teaspoon garlic, minced
⅛ teaspoon sweet paprika
¼ teaspoon chili powder
Salt and pepper to taste

Method:
In a medium nonstick sauté pan heat the oil. Add turkey, onion, vinegar, garlic, paprika, and salt and pepper. Sauté until cooked through. In a medium bowl combine Zoned Pepper Relish, apple, and chili powder. Spoon relish onto serving plate and top with turkey.

TURKEY SCALOPPINI WITH MUSHROOMS

Servings: 1 Dinner Entrée (4 blocks)

Block Size:	**Ingredients:**
4 Protein	4 ounces turkey breast, sliced in strips
½ Carbohydrate	½ cup onion, finely chopped
1 Carbohydrate	3 cups mushrooms, thinly sliced
2 Carbohydrate	⅔ cup unsweetened applesauce
½ Carbohydrate	2 teaspoons cornstarch
4 Fat	1⅓ teaspoons olive oil, divided

Spices:

2 teaspoons cider vinegar
1 teaspoon orange extract
⅛ teaspoon dill
¼ teaspoon cinnamon
1 cup lemon- and lime-flavored water
⅛ teaspoon lemon herb seasoning

Method:

Heat ⅔ teaspoon oil in medium nonstick sauté pan. Sauté turkey with onion, cider vinegar, and lemon herb seasoning. Sauté until turkey is cooked through, about 1 to 2 minutes. In second sauté pan heat remaining oil and sauté mushrooms for 3 to 5 minutes. Add remaining ingredients and sauté until liquid is thickened. (Mix cornstarch with a little water to dissolve it before adding to saucepan.) Spoon mushroom mixture onto serving plate and top with turkey.

TURKEY WITH LENTILS AND SPINACH

Servings: 1 Dinner Entrée (4 blocks)

Block Size:	Ingredients:
4 Protein	6 ounces lean ground turkey
¼ Carbohydrate	½ cup celery, chopped
¼ Carbohydrate	¼ cup onion, chopped
1 Carbohydrate	½ cup Zoned Italian Sauce (see page 150)
½ Carbohydrate	3 cups spinach, chopped
2 Carbohydrate	½ cup cooked lentils
4 Fat	1⅓ teaspoons olive oil

Spices:

1 teaspoon garlic, chopped
1 tablespoon fresh parsley, chopped
Dash fresh grated nutmeg
Salt and pepper to taste

Method:

Heat oil in a medium nonstick sauté pan. Add turkey, celery, onion, garlic, parsley, nutmeg, salt and pepper. Cook until turkey is cooked through and vegetables are slightly softened. Stir in Zoned Italian Sauce, lentils, and spinach. Heat through and spoon into a medium serving bowl.

CORDON BLEU CHICKEN STUFFED WITH HAM

Servings: 1 Dinner Entrée (4 blocks)

Block Size:	Ingredients:
3 Protein	3 ounces chicken breast (boneless, skinless)
½ Protein	¾ ounce deli-style ham, diced
½ Protein	½ ounce low-fat Swiss cheese
1 Carbohydrate	1 cup leeks, sliced (white part only)
1 Carbohydrate	¾ cup Zoned Espagnol (Brown) Sauce (see page 155)
½ Carbohydrate	1 cup celery, sliced
½ Carbohydrate	1½ cups mushrooms, quartered
1 Carbohydrate	1 cup green beans, 2-inch pieces
4 Fat	1⅓ teaspoons olive oil, divided

Spices:

⅛ teaspoon dried thyme
¼ teaspoon parsley, chopped
Salt and pepper to taste

Method:

Flatten chicken breast until ¼-inch thick. Place ham and cheese in the center of the flattened chicken breast and sprinkle with thyme, parsley, salt and pepper. Roll up chicken breast around filling and secure with toothpicks. Brush ⅓ teaspoon oil onto a baking dish. Place rolled chicken in dish and cover tightly. Bake in a preheated 350-degree Fahrenheit oven for 15 to 20 minutes. Heat remaining oil in a medium nonstick sauté pan, then add leeks, celery, mushrooms, and green beans and cook for 3 to 5 minutes. When the vegetables are tender blend in Zoned Espagnol Sauce and heat through. Spoon vegetables onto serving plate and top with rolled chicken breast.

SOUTHWESTERN CHICKEN WITH PEPPER AND BEAN SALSA

Servings: 1 Dinner Entrée (4 blocks)

Block Size:	Ingredients:
4 Protein	4 ounces chicken tenderloin, diced
1 Carbohydrate	½ cup salsa*
½ Carbohydrate	½ cup onion, chopped
1 Carbohydrate	¼ cup kidney beans, rinsed
½ Carbohydrate	3 cups spinach
1 Carbohydrate	¼ cup black beans, rinsed
4 Fat	1⅓ teaspoons olive oil

Spices:

1 tablespoon garlic, minced
⅛ teaspoon celery salt
2 teaspoons chili powder
Black pepper to taste

Method:

Heat oil in a medium nonstick sauté pan and add chicken and garlic. Sauté until chicken is cooked through and slightly browned. Add salsa, onion, kidney beans, black beans, chili powder, celery salt, and pepper and heat through. Form spinach into a bed on serving plate. Top with chicken mixture and serve.

*Note: We used a medium-heat salsa. Use whatever strength you prefer.

SPICY TOFU WITH SCALLIONS AND RADISHES

Servings: 1 Dinner Entrée (4 blocks)

Block Size:	Ingredients:
4 Protein	12 ounces extra-firm tofu, 1-inch cubes
1 Carbohydrate	1½ cups jalapeño and red bell pepper, finely diced (mixed to desired heat)
½ Carbohydrate	2 cups fresh spinach, torn
¼ Carbohydrate	½ cup radishes, thinly sliced
1 Carbohydrate	1 cup tomatoes, seeded and diced
½ Carbohydrate	½ cup scallions, chopped
¾ Carbohydrate	¾ cup canned mushroom slices
4 Fat	1⅓ teaspoons olive oil

Spices:

1 tablespoon lemon juice
1 tablespoon water
4 teaspoons soy sauce
½ tablespoon white wine
¾ teaspoon gingerroot, minced
¼ teaspoon garlic, minced
Salt and pepper to taste

Method:
Heat oil and ¼ teaspoon gingerroot in medium sauté pan. Stir-fry tofu until browned on all sides. Whisk lemon juice, water, soy sauce, wine, garlic, salt, pepper, and remaining gingerroot together in a small bowl. Combine vegetables in a medium bowl and pour in soy sauce mixture. Toss to coat. Add in tofu and spoon onto serving dish.

MUSHROOM TENDERLOIN WITH ARTICHOKE HEARTS

Servings: 1 Dinner Entrée (4 blocks)

Block Size:	Ingredients:
4 Protein	4 ounces beef tenderloin
1 Carbohydrate	1 cup Zoned Mushroom Sauce (see page 148)
1 Carbohydrate	1 cup onions, chopped
2 Carbohydrate	6 small artichoke hearts, diced*
4 Fat	1⅓ teaspoons olive oil

Method:

In a nonstick sauté pan sauté add oil, onion, artichoke hearts, and beef. Cook until beef is done and vegetables are tender. Add Zoned Mushroom Sauce and heat through. Place mixture on a large dinner plate and serve immediately.

*Note: 3 small artichoke hearts equal 1 medium artichoke.

ITALIAN-STYLE STEAK AND PEPPERS

Servings: 1 Dinner Entrée (4 blocks)

Block Size:	Ingredients:
3 Protein	3 ounces lean beef
1 Protein	1 ounce skim milk mozzarella, shredded
1 Carbohydrate	½ cup Zoned Italian Sauce (see page 150)
2 Carbohydrate	2¼ cups red and green pepper strips
1 Carbohydrate	1 cup onion, diced
4 Fat	1⅓ teaspoons olive oil

Method:

In a nonstick sauté pan, place oil, beef, and vegetables. Cook until beef is done and vegetables are tender. Add Zoned Italian Sauce and heat through. Top with cheese and serve.

CONDIMENTS AND SAUCES

ZONED MUSHROOM SAUCE

Servings: Four 1-cup servings, 1 Carbohydrate Block each*

Block Size:	Ingredients:
1½ Carbohydrate	4½ cups mushrooms, sliced
2½ Carbohydrate	10 teaspoons cornstarch

Spices:

3 cups strong beef stock
⅛ teaspoon Worcestershire sauce
1 tablespoon red wine
⅛ teaspoon chili powder
½ teaspoon garlic, chopped
1 tablespoon dried parsley flakes
Salt and pepper to taste

Method:
Combine all ingredients in a small saucepan to form a sauce. (Mix cornstarch with a little cold water to dissolve it before adding to saucepan.) Heat sauce to a simmer, constantly stirring until mixture thickens. Transfer sauce mixture to a storage container, let cool, and refrigerate.** Each time you make a Zone-favorable meal use this sauce as a replacement for 1 Carbohydrate Zone Block.

*Note: Each cup of Zoned Mushroom Sauce contains 1 Carbohydrate Zone Block. There are no Protein or Fat Blocks in this sauce recipe. This recipe is used as a component in other Zone Recipes.

**Note: This sauce may be refrigerated for up to 5 days, or if you prefer the sauce may be frozen and defrosted for later use. Although the sauce is freeze-thaw stable, after sauce has been frozen and defrosted it may need to be stirred to reincorporate the small amount of moisture that forms on the sauce during the freezing and thawing process.

ZONED COUNTRY-STYLE CHICKEN GRAVY

Servings: Four 1-cup servings, 1 Carbohydrate Block each*

Block Size:	**Ingredients:**
2 Carbohydrate	2 cups onions, sliced
2 Carbohydrate	8 teaspoons cornstarch

Spices:

2½ cups strong chicken stock
1 tablespoon white wine
½ teaspoon garlic, chopped
½ teaspoon celery salt
1 teaspoon dried parsley flakes
Salt and pepper to taste

Method:

Combine all ingredients in a small saucepan to form a sauce. (Mix cornstarch with a little cold water to dissolve it before adding to saucepan.) Heat sauce to a simmer, constantly stirring until mixture thickens. Transfer sauce mixture to a storage container, let cool and refrigerate.** Each time you make a Zone-favorable meal use this sauce as a replacement for 1 Carbohydrate Zone Block.

*Note: Each cup of Zoned Country-Style Chicken Gravy contains 1 Carbohydrate Zone Block. There are no Protein or Fat Blocks in this sauce recipe. This recipe is used as a component in other Zone Recipes.

**Note: This sauce may be refrigerated for up to 5 days, or if you prefer the sauce may be frozen and defrosted for later use. Although the sauce is freeze-thaw stable, after sauce has been frozen and defrosted it may need to be stirred to reincorporate the small amount of moisture that forms on the sauce during the freezing and thawing process.

ZONED ITALIAN SAUCE

Servings: Four ½-cup servings, 1 Carbohydrate Block each*

Block Size:	Ingredients:
3 Carbohydrate	1½ cups tomato puree
1 Carbohydrate	4 teaspoons cornstarch

Spices:

1 cup strong chicken stock
1 tablespoon red wine
1 teaspoon dried parsley flakes
1 teaspoon dried oregano
1 teaspoon dried basil
⅛ teaspoon ground dried thyme
⅛ teaspoon ground nutmeg
1½ teaspoon garlic, chopped

Method:
Combine all ingredients in a small saucepan to form a sauce. (Mix cornstarch with a little cold water to dissolve it before adding to saucepan.) Heat sauce to a simmer, constantly stirring with a whip until mixture thickens. Transfer sauce mixture to a storage container, let cool, and refrigerate.** Each time you make a Zone-favorable meal use this sauce as a replacement for 1 Carbohydrate Zone Block.

*Note: Each ½ cup of Zoned Italian Sauce contains 1 Carbohydrate Zone Block. There is no Protein or Fat Blocks in this sauce recipe. This recipe is used as a component in other Zone Recipes.

**Note: This sauce may be refrigerated for up to 5 days, or if you prefer the sauce may be frozen and defrosted for later use. Although the sauce is freeze-thaw stable, after sauce has been frozen and defrosted it may need to be stirred to reincorporate the small amount of moisture that forms on the sauce during the freezing and thawing process.

ZONED WHITE SAUCE

*Servings: Four ½-cup servings, 1 Protein Block and
1 Carbohydrate Block each**

Block Size:	Ingredients:
1 Protein	1 envelope Knox unflavored gelatin
1 Protein	1 ounce white low-fat cheddar cheese, shredded
2 Protein and 2 Carbohydrate	2 cups 1 percent milk
1½ Carbohydrate	6 teaspoons cornstarch
½ Carbohydrate	½ cup onion, finely minced or pureed in a blender

Spices:

½ cup low-fat chicken stock
⅛ teaspoon celery salt
⅛ teaspoon Worcestershire sauce
White pepper to taste

Method:

Combine all ingredients in a small non-aluminum saucepan to form a sauce. (Mix cornstarch with a little cold water to dissolve it before adding to saucepan.) Heat sauce to a simmer, constantly stirring with a whip until mixture thickens. Transfer sauce mixture to a storage container, let cool, and refrigerate.** Each time you make a Zone-favorable meal use this sauce as a replacement for 1 Carbohydrate Zone Block.

*Note: Each ½ cup of Zoned White Sauce contains 1 Protein Zone Block and 1 Carbohydrate Zone Block. There are no Fat Blocks in this sauce recipe. This recipe is used as a component in other Zone Recipes.

**Note: This sauce may be refrigerated for up to 5 days, or if you prefer the sauce may be frozen and defrosted for later use. Although the sauce is

freeze-thaw stable, after sauce has been frozen and defrosted it may need to be stirred to reincorporate the small amount of moisture that forms on the sauce during the freezing and thawing process.

ZONED FINE HERB CHEESE SAUCE

Servings: Four ½-cup servings, 1 Protein Block and 1 Carbohydrate Block each*

Block Size:	Ingredients:
2 Protein	2 ounces yellow low-fat cheddar cheese
2 Protein and 2 Carbohydrate	2 cups 1 percent milk
1½ Carbohydrate	6 teaspoons cornstarch
½ Carbohydrate	½ cup onion, finely minced or pureed in a blender

Spices:

½ tablespoon dry sherry
⅛ teaspoon dried parsley
⅛ teaspoon dried chives
⅛ teaspoon dried basil
1 teaspoon paprika
⅛ teaspoon chili powder
⅛ teaspoon Worcestershire sauce
⅛ teaspoon celery salt
1 teaspoon garlic, minced
½ teaspoon lemon herb seasoning

Method:
Combine all ingredients in a small non-aluminum saucepan to form a sauce. (Mix cornstarch with a little cold water to dissolve it before adding

to saucepan.) Heat sauce to a simmer, constantly stirring with a whip until mixture thickens. Transfer sauce mixture to a storage container, let cool, and refrigerate.** Each time you make a Zone-favorable meal use this sauce as a replacement for 1 Carbohydrate Zone Block.

Note: Each ½ cup of Zoned Fine Herb Cheese Sauce contains 1 Protein Zone Block and 1 Carbohydrate Zone Block. There are no Fat Blocks in this sauce recipe. This recipe is used as a component in other Zone Recipes.

**Note: This sauce may be refrigerated for up to 5 days, or if you prefer the sauce may be frozen and defrosted for later use. Although the sauce is freeze-thaw stable, after sauce has been frozen and defrosted it may need to be stirred to reincorporate the small amount of moisture that forms on the sauce during the freezing and thawing process.*

ZONED BARBECUE SAUCE

Servings: Four ½-cup servings, 1 Carbohydrate Block each*

Block Size:

1 Carbohydrate
2 Carbohydrate
1 Carbohydrate

Ingredients:

4 teaspoons cornstarch
1 cup tomato puree
⅓ cup unsweetened applesauce

Spices:

1 tablespoon liquid smoke flavoring
4 teaspoons garlic, minced
1 teaspoon Worcestershire sauce
¾ cup strong chicken stock
3 tablespoons cider vinegar
¼ teaspoon chili powder

Method:
Combine all ingredients in a small saucepan to form a sauce. (Mix cornstarch with a little cold water to dissolve it before adding to saucepan.) Heat sauce to a simmer, constantly stirring with a whip until mixture thickens. Transfer sauce mixture to a storage container, let cool, and refrigerate.** Each time you make a Zone-favorable meal use this sauce as a replacement for 1 Carbohydrate Zone Block.

*Note: Each ½ cup of Zoned Barbecue Sauce contains 1 Carbohydrate Zone Block. There are no Protein or Fat Blocks in this sauce recipe. This recipe is used as a component in other Zone Recipes.

**Note: This sauce may be refrigerated for up to 5 days, or if you prefer the sauce may be frozen and defrosted for later use. Although the sauce is freeze-thaw stable, after sauce has been frozen and defrosted it may need to be stirred to reincorporate the small amount of moisture that forms on the sauce during the freezing and thawing process.

ZONED ESPAGNOL (BROWN) SAUCE

Servings: Four ¾-cup servings, 1 Carbohydrate Block each*

Block Size:

1 Carbohydrate
¼ Carbohydrate
2¾ Carbohydrate

Ingredients:

½ cup tomato puree
¼ cup onion, finely diced
11 teaspoons cornstarch

Spices:

3 cups strong beef stock
⅛ teaspoon Worcestershire sauce
1 tablespoon red wine
2 teaspoons garlic, chopped
⅛ teaspoon dried oregano
1 teaspoon dried parsley flakes
Salt and pepper to taste

Method:

Combine all ingredients in a small saucepan to form a sauce. (Mix cornstarch with a little cold water to dissolve it before adding to saucepan.) Heat sauce to a simmer, constantly stirring with a whip until mixture thickens. Transfer sauce mixture to a storage container, let cool, and refrigerate.** Each time you make a Zone-favorable meal use this sauce as a replacement for 1 Carbohydrate Zone Block.

*Note: Each ¾ cup of Zoned Espagnol (Brown) Sauce contains 1 Carbohydrate Zone Block. There are no Protein or Fat Blocks in this sauce recipe. This recipe is used as a component in other Zone Recipes.

**Note: This sauce may be refrigerated for up to 5 days, or if you prefer the sauce may be frozen and defrosted for later use. Although the sauce is freeze-thaw stable, after sauce has been frozen and defrosted it may need to be stirred to reincorporate the small amount of moisture that forms on the sauce during the freezing and thawing process.

ZONED HERB DRESSING

Servings: Four ½-cup servings, 1 Carbohydrate Block each*

Block Size:	Ingredients:
1 Carbohydrate	1 cup onion, finely minced
1 Carbohydrate	¼ cup chickpeas, canned, minced finely
2 Carbohydrate	8 teaspoons cornstarch

Spices:

1¾ cups water
¼ cup cider vinegar
2 tablespoons balsamic vinegar
⅛ teaspoon Worcestershire sauce
1 teaspoon dried tarragon
1 teaspoon dried oregano
1 teaspoon parsley flakes
2 teaspoons garlic, minced
1 teaspoon dried basil
⅛ teaspoon chili powder
½ teaspoon celery salt
1 teaspoon dried dill

Method:

Combine all ingredients in a small saucepan to form a thickened dressing. (Mix cornstarch with a little cold water to dissolve it before adding to saucepan.) Heat dressing to a simmer, constantly stirring until mixture thickens. Transfer dressing mixture to a storage container, let cool, and refrigerate.** Each time you make a Zone-favorable meal use this dressing as a replacement for 1 Carbohydrate Zone Block.

*Note: Each ½ cup of Zoned Herb Dressing contains 1 Carbohydrate Zone Block. There are no Protein or Fat Blocks in this sauce recipe. This recipe is used as a component in other Zone Recipes.

**Note:* This dressing may be refrigerated for up to 5 days, or if you prefer the dressing may be frozen and defrosted for later use. Although the dressing is freeze-thaw stable, after dressing has been frozen and defrosted it may need to be stirred to reincorporate the small amount of moisture that forms on the dressing during the freezing and thawing process.*

ZONED FRENCH DRESSING

*Servings: Four ½-cup servings, 1 Carbohydrate Block each**

Block Size:

½ Carbohydrate
½ Carbohydrate
2 Carbohydrate
1 Carbohydrate

Ingredients:

½ cup onion, finely minced
¼ cup tomato puree
8 teaspoons cornstarch
¼ cup kidney beans, canned, rinsed, and minced

Spices:

1¾ cups water
¼ cup cider vinegar
2 tablespoons balsamic vinegar
⅛ teaspoon Worcestershire sauce
1 teaspoon dried tarragon
1 teaspoon dried oregano
1 teaspoon dried parsley flakes
3 teaspoons garlic, minced
1 teaspoon dried basil
½ teaspoon chili powder
2 teaspoons paprika
1 teaspoon dried dill

Method:
Combine all ingredients in a small saucepan to form a thickened dressing. (Mix cornstarch with a little cold water to dissolve it before

adding to saucepan.) Heat dressing to a simmer, constantly stirring until mixture thickens. Let dressing cool for about 10 to 15 minutes, then place dressing in a food processor and blend for 2 to 3 minutes until a smooth consistency forms. Transfer dressing mixture to a storage container, let cool, and refrigerate.** Each time you make a Zone-favorable meal use this dressing as a replacement for 1 Carbohydrate Zone Block.

*Note: Each ½ cup of Zoned French Dressing contains 1 Carbohydrate Zone Block. There are no Protein or Fat Blocks in this sauce recipe. This recipe is used as a component in other Zone Recipes.

**Note: This dressing may be refrigerated for up to 5 days, or if you prefer, the dressing may be frozen and defrosted for later use. Although the dressing is freeze-thaw stable, after dressing has been frozen and defrosted it may need to be stirred to reincorporate the small amount of moisture that forms on the dressing during the freezing and thawing process.

ZONED PEPPER RELISH

Servings: Four ¾-cup servings, 1 Carbohydrate Block each*

Block Size:	Ingredients:
1½ Carbohydrate	3½ cups frozen red and green bell pepper strips
½ Carbohydrate	½ cup frozen onions, chopped
1 Carbohydrate	½ cup tomato puree
½ Carbohydrate	½ cup tomato, chopped
½ Carbohydrate	2 teaspoons cornstarch

Spices:

¼ cup water
1 tablespoon cider vinegar
2 teaspoons pickling spice
½ teaspoon lemon herb seasoning
⅛ teaspoon celery salt

Method:

Combine all ingredients in a small saucepan to form the pepper relish. (Mix cornstarch with a little cold water to dissolve it before adding to saucepan.) Heat relish to a simmer, constantly stirring until mixture thickens. Simmer for 3 to 5 minutes until entire mixture is hot. Transfer relish mixture to a storage container, let cool, and refrigerate.** Each time you make a Zone-favorable meal use this dressing as a replacement for 1 Carbohydrate Zone Block.

*Note: Each ¾ cup of Zoned Pepper Relish contains 1 Carbohydrate Zone Block. There are no Protein or Fat Blocks in this sauce recipe. This recipe is used as a component in other Zone Recipes or used as a condiment to other Zone Recipes.

**Note: This relish may be refrigerated for up to 5 days, or if you prefer the relish may be frozen and defrosted for later use. Although the relish is freeze-thaw stable, after relish has been frozen and defrosted it may need to be stirred to reincorporate the small amount of moisture that forms on the relish during the freezing and thawing process.

ZONED TARRAGON MUSTARD SAUCE

Servings: Four ½-cup servings, 1 Carbohydrate Block each*

Block Size: **Ingredients:**

2 Carbohydrate   ½ cup chickpeas, canned, minced
                            finely

2 Carbohydrate   8 teaspoons cornstarch

Spices:

2 cups chicken stock
2 tablespoons cider vinegar
½ teaspoon Worcestershire sauce
2 teaspoons dried tarragon
2 teaspoons ground mustard
¼ teaspoon turmeric
2 teaspoons garlic, minced

Method:

Combine all ingredients in a small saucepan to form a sauce. (Mix cornstarch with a little cold water to dissolve it before adding to saucepan.) Heat sauce to a simmer, constantly stirring with a whip until mixture thickens. Transfer sauce mixture to a storage container, let cool, and refrigerate.** Each time you make a Zone-favorable meal use this sauce as a replacement for 1 Carbohydrate Zone Block.

*Note: Each ½ cup of Zoned Tarragon Mustard Sauce contains 1 Carbohydrate Zone Block. There are no Protein or Fat Blocks in this sauce recipe. This recipe is used as a component in other Zone Recipes.

**Note: This sauce may be refrigerated for up to 5 days, or if you prefer the sauce may be frozen and defrosted for later use. Although the sauce is freeze-thaw stable, after sauce has been frozen and defrosted it may need to be stirred to reincorporate the small amount of moisture that forms on the sauce during the freezing and thawing process.

ZONED CHINESE PICKLED VEGETABLES

Servings: Four ½-cup, 1 Carbohydrate Block each*

Block Size:

Ingredients:

1 Carbohydrate   1½ cups frozen broccoli florets

1 Carbohydrate   ⅓ cup canned water chestnuts, sliced

1 Carbohydrate   2 teaspoons sugar

½ Carbohydrate   1½ cups cabbage, shredded (or coleslaw mix)

½ Carbohydrate   1 cup frozen cauliflower florets

Spices:

1 teaspoon garlic, minced

1 tablespoon Worcestershire sauce

1 tablespoon soy sauce

¼ teaspoon celery salt

1 teaspoon pickling spice

2 cups water

⅛ teaspoon hot red pepper flakes (optional)

Method: Combine all ingredients in a saucepan and bring to a boil. Reduce heat and simmer for 10 minutes. Transfer mixture to a storage container, let cool, and refrigerate. Each time you make a Zone-favorable meal use these pickled vegetables as a replacement for 1 Carbohydrate Zone Block.

*Note: Each ½ cup of Zoned Chinese Pickled Vegetables contains 1 Carbohydrate Zone Block. There are no Protein or Fat Blocks in this sauce recipe. This recipe is used as a component in other Zone Recipes.

DESSERTS AND SNACKS

FROZEN YOGURT ALASKA JUBILEE

Servings: 8 Serving Dishes (1 block each)

Block Size:	Ingredients:
3 Protein	3 envelopes Knox unflavored gelatin
1 Protein	2 egg whites, uncooked
4 Protein and	
4 Carbohydrate	2 cups plain low-fat yogurt
3 Carbohydrate	1½ cups canned pitted tart cherries, in water
1 Carbohydrate	2 teaspoons sugar
8 Fat	8 teaspoons almonds, slivered and toasted

Spices:

2 teaspoons cherry extract
½ teaspoon vanilla extract
⅛ teaspoon powdered ginger

Method:

In saucepan, combine yogurt, gelatin, fruit, extracts, and ginger. Heat until mixture becomes thoroughly warm, no more than 180 degrees. Set aside yogurt mixture and let cool. In a mixing bowl, whip egg whites and sugar until firm. When the mixture in the saucepan has cooled, combine mixture with whipped egg whites and chopped almonds. Place mixture in a pan and place in freezer or add mixture to an ice cream maker and blend. When mixture is frozen, scoop into eight small serving dishes.

HOMEMADE CINNAMON APPLESAUCE
WITH YOGURT

Servings: 8 Serving Dishes (1 block each)

Block Size:	Ingredients:
4 Protein	4 envelopes Knox unflavored gelatin
4 Protein and 4 Carbohydrate	2 cups plain low-fat yogurt
4 Carbohydrate	2 Granny Smith apples, cored and diced in ½-inch cubes
8 Fat	8 teaspoons almonds, slivered and toasted

Spices:

1 teaspoon ground cinnamon
½ teaspoon pure lemon extract

Method:

In a medium bowl, combine yogurt, gelatin, fruit, almonds, cinnamon, and extract. Blend well, chill, and serve in 8 serving bowls.

POACHED PEAR WITH CHEESE

Servings: 8 Serving Dishes (1 block each)

Block Size:	Ingredients:
8 Protein	2 cups low-fat cottage cheese
6 Carbohydrate	3 pears, halved, cored, and sliced in thin strips
1 Carbohydrate	4 ounces Johannesburg Riesling
½ Carbohydrate	2 teaspoons cornstarch
½ Carbohydrate	¼ cup blueberries
8 Fat	8 teaspoons almonds, slivered

Spices:

½ teaspoon orange extract
½ teaspoon lemon extract
Dash of ground cloves

Method:

In a small nonstick sauté pan, combine wine, extracts, and cornstarch. (Mix cornstarch in wine before adding to sauté pan.) Add pears to the sauté pan and bring to a simmer. Simmer for 3 to 5 minutes, stirring frequently, until the pears soften and the juices reduce and thicken. As the mixture cooks add cloves. Divide cottage cheese into the bottom of 8 serving bowls. Place warm pears on top of cottage cheese. Sprinkle with almonds and blueberries and serve.

PEACHES WITH A AND A TOPPING

Servings: 8 Serving Dishes (1 block each)

Block Size:	Ingredients:
8 Protein	2 cups low-fat cottage cheese
4½ Carbohydrate	4½ peaches, halved and pitted
2 Carbohydrate	⅔ cup unsweetened applesauce
½ Carbohydrate	2 teaspoons cornstarch
1 Carbohydrate	4 ounces Johannesburg Riesling
8 Fat	8 teaspoons almonds, finely chopped

Spices:

2 tablespoons water
½ teaspoon orange extract
½ teaspoon lemon extract
Dash ground cloves
⅛ teaspoon ground ginger
Dash ground cinnamon

Method:
In a small nonstick sauté pan, combine wine, water, extracts, cloves, ginger, and cornstarch. (Mix cornstarch in wine before adding to sauté pan.) Add peaches to the sauté pan and bring to a simmer. Simmer for 3 to 5 minutes, stirring frequently, until the peaches soften and the juices reduce and thicken. In a small bowl whip together applesauce, almonds, and cinnamon. Divide cottage cheese into the bottom of 8 serving bowls. Place warm peaches on top of cottage cheese. Spoon on almonds and applesauce topping and serve.

GLAZED SPICED APPLE

Servings: 4 Serving Dishes (1 block each)

Block Size:	Ingredients:
4 Protein	4 ounces low-fat cheddar cheese, shredded
2 Carbohydrate	1 red Delicious apple, cored and cut into 1-inch cubes
1 Carbohydrate	1 peach, halved, pitted, and finely diced
½ Carbohydrate	1 teaspoon brown sugar
½ Carbohydrate	2 teaspoons cornstarch
4 Fat	4 teaspoons almonds, sliced and toasted

Spices:

½ cup water
3 tablespoons cider vinegar
¼ teaspoon lemon extract
⅛ teaspoon ground cinnamon
Dash celery salt

Method:
Combine all ingredients (except cheese) in a small saucepan. Stirring constantly, over medium heat, cook until the apple is thoroughly coated and a sauce forms. Continue simmering 3 to 5 minutes until flavors are blended. Spoon into bowls, top with shredded cheese, and serve hot.

SHRIMP AND VEGETABLE PLATTER

Servings: 4 Serving Dishes (1 block each)

Block Size:	Ingredients:
4 Protein	6 ounces baby shrimp
1 Carbohydrate	2 cups broccoli florets
1 Carbohydrate	1 cup celery, julienne
1 Carbohydrate	1 cup cherry tomatoes
1 Carbohydrate	½ cup Zoned Herb Dressing (see page 156)
4 Fat	12 black olives

Method:

Place Zoned Herb Dressing into 4 small serving dishes, and place on center of 4 serving plates. Arrange an equal amount of vegetables, olives, and shrimp around the edge of each plate.

BLUSHING PEAR

Servings: 8 Serving Dishes (1 block each)

Block Size:	Ingredients:
8 Protein	8 ounces low-fat cottage cheese
6 Carbohydrate	3 pears, cored, halved, and sliced into thin strips
1 Carbohydrate	4 ounces white Zinfandel
½ Carbohydrate	2 teaspoons cornstarch
½ Carbohydrate	½ cup raspberries
8 Fat	8 teaspoons almonds, finely chopped

Spices:

½ teaspoon orange extract
½ teaspoon lemon extract
Dash of ground cloves

Method:

In a small nonstick sauté pan, combine wine, extracts, and cornstarch. (Mix cornstarch in wine before adding to sauté pan.) Add pears to the sauté pan and bring to a simmer. Simmer for 3 to 5 minutes, stirring frequently, until the pears soften and the juices reduce and thicken. As the mixture cooks, add cloves. Divide cottage cheese into the bottom of 8 serving bowls. Place warm pears on top of cottage cheese. Sprinkle with raspberries and almonds and serve.

BLUEBERRY CUSTARD JUBILEE

Servings: 4 Serving Dishes (1 block each)

Block Size:

2 Protein
2 Protein and
2 Carbohydrate

1 Carbohydrate
1 Carbohydrate

Ingredients:

2 whole eggs

2 cups 1 percent milk

½ cup blueberries
2 teaspoons sugar

Spices:

⅛ teaspoon vanilla extract or lemon zest

Method:

Beat eggs until they are light and fluffy; then put eggs, milk, vanilla extract, and sugar in a nonstick saucepan. Heat mixture to a simmer, but not boiling. Pour mixture into 4 serving dishes and refrigerator to cool. After mixture has cooled for 20 minutes divide blueberries into 4 serving dishes and return to refrigerator. Serve when custard has set.

TANGY FRUIT FLUFF

Servings: 4 Serving Dishes (1 block each)

Block Size:	Ingredients:
3 Protein	6 egg whites
1 Protein	1 envelope Knox unflavored gelatin
2 Carbohydrate	1 cup blueberries
1 Carbohydrate	1 cup raspberries
1 Carbohydrate	¾ cup blackberries

Method:

In a mixing bowl whip egg whites and gelatin until a fluffy mixture with stiff peaks forms. Slowly fold berries into whipped egg whites. Equally divide mixture into 4 serving dishes and sprinkle with almonds. Place serving dishes in freezer until set.

MELON SMOOTHIE

Servings: 4 Glasses (1 block each)

Block Size:	Ingredients:
1 Protein	⅓ ounce protein powder
2 Protein and 2 Carbohydrate	2 cups 1 percent milk
1 Protein and 1 Carbohydrate	½ cup plain low-fat yogurt
1 Carbohydrate	¾ cup cantaloupe chunks
4 Fat	4 teaspoons almonds, slivered

Method:

Place all ingredients except protein powder in blender. Blend until smooth, then add protein powder. Pour into four glasses and serve immediately.

RASPBERRY-LIME SMOOTHIE

Servings: 4 Glasses (1 block each)

Block Size:	Ingredients:
2 Protein	⅔ ounce protein powder
1 Protein and	
1 Carbohydrate	1 cup 1 percent milk
1 Protein and	
1 Carbohydrate	½ cup plain low-fat yogurt
1 Carbohydrate	1 cup raspberries
1 Carbohydrate	Juice of 1 lime
4 Fat	4 teaspoons almonds, slivered

Method:
Place all ingredients except protein powder in blender. Blend until smooth, then add protein powder. Pour into four glasses and serve immediately.

STRAWBERRY-ORANGE SMOOTHIE

Servings: 4 Glasses (1 block each)

Block Size:	Ingredients:
2 Protein	⅔ ounce protein powder
1 Protein and	
1 Carbohydrate	1 cup 1 percent milk
1 Protein and	
1 Carbohydrate	½ cup plain low-fat yogurt
1 Carbohydrate	1 cup strawberries
1 Carbohydrate	⅓ cup Mandarin orange segments
4 Fat	4 teaspoons almonds, slivered

Method:

Place all ingredients except protein powder in blender. Blend until smooth, then add protein powder. Pour into four glasses and serve immediately.

ZONE-PERFECT GOURMET MEALS

Let's face it. Gourmet meals are called gourmet meals because they are difficult to prepare and take more time to present. But there will be those occasions when you will want to take the time to prepare a gourmet meal, and of course you want to make it Zone-Perfect.

Fortunately, some of the best chefs in America have already done the work for you. This meal comes from La Bocage, which is one of the top French restaurants in the Greater Boston area. For a recent meeting of the Boston Culinary Society, Susanna Harwell-Tolini and Ed Tolini prepared the following Zone meal, consisting of chicken consommé with chicken quenelles, poached Atlantic salmon with asparagus coulis, baked tomatoes stuffed with spinach using a tomato sauce, and strawberry mousse. Here's how to make this gourmet Zone meal for a party of six:

CHICKEN STOCK

Ingredients:

1 large stewing fowl
1½–2 gallons cold water
1 cup carrots (diced)
1 cup onions (diced)
1 cup celery (diced)
1 cup leeks (diced)
¼ cup loosely packed fresh parsley
2 bay leaves
1 teaspoon thyme

Method:
In a large pot, place the stewing fowl and cover with cold water; then add the vegetables and herbs. Bring the water to a boil, and skim off the fat and impurities. Add the spices and simmer 4 to 5 hours. Strain the broth and cool, then refrigerate.

CHICKEN CONSOMMÉ

Ingredients:

1½ quarts chilled chicken stock
½ cup carrots (coarsely chopped)
½ cup onions (coarsely chopped)
½ cup fresh tomato (chopped)
½ cup egg whites (lightly beaten)
½ pound chicken meat (ground skinless chicken breast with no fat)
2 bay leaves
2 sprigs fresh thyme
1 teaspoon black peppercorns (crushed)
1 teaspoon salt

Method:
Puree the vegetables in a food processor fitted with a steel blade. Combine the vegetables with the ground chicken meat and mix with the lightly beaten egg whites. Add the herbs and seasonings. Marinate and chill for 1 hour. Place the ingredients in a stockpot with the chilled chicken stock. Stir well to incorporate. Stir until the stock has come to a slow boil. Simmer 2 to 3 hours. The raft should be well formed on the top of the consommé.* Do not boil rapidly, as this will cause the raft to break and fall. After simmering, strain through a fine strainer with cheesecloth. Serve with chicken quenelles (see following page) in a warmed soup bowl.

Note: A raft is the culinary term used to describe the solid mass formed by the vegetables, egg whites, and spices to remove impurities from stock.

CHICKEN QUENELLES

Ingredients:

8 ounces skinless chicken breast
1 tablespoon egg whites
2 teaspoons light cream
2 ounces chicken stock
½ nutmeg (freshly ground)
1 pint chicken broth
Salt and white pepper to taste

Method:

Puree chicken breast in a food processor. Add the light cream, egg whites, and 2 ounces chicken broth while the processor is on. Be sure to emulsify all of the liquid ingredients into the chicken. Season with salt, pepper, and nutmeg. Heat the pint of chicken broth in a small pan to boiling point. Test one or two quenelles for flavor and texture by dropping a small ball of the chicken mixture in the stock. Taste and correct the seasonings if needed. Cook the remaining quenelles by taking soupspoons and dropping round or oval shapes into the stock (about 2 full teaspoons each). Serve 1½ ounces per person.

POACHED ATLANTIC SALMON WITH ASPARAGUS COULIS

Servings: 6

Ingredients:

6 each 4½-ounce Atlantic salmon fillets (skins removed)
1 bunch asparagus (peeled and stems removed)

Court Bouillon:

1 quart water
1 cup dry white wine
1 small white onion, peeled
½ cup leek greens, diced
2 ribs celery
3 large bay leaves
1 teaspoon black peppercorns
½ cup parsley stems

Asparagus Coulis (may need additional asparagus for the coulis):

3 large shallots, peeled and cut in quarters
1 large white leek (diced)
¾ cup chicken stock
1 pound asparagus trimmings (stems and reserved peelings)
1 cup chicken stock
¼ bunch sorrel
¼ bunch watercress

Method:

Peel and cut the woody stems from the asparagus. Reserve the peelings and stems. Blanch the asparagus in boiling water. Immediately cool and reserve for final presentation. Combine the ingredients for the court bouillon in a medium skillet or saucepan and simmer for 45 minutes.

For the Coulis:

Simmer the shallots and leek white in the ¾ cup of chicken stock for 20 minutes. Add the asparagus trimmings and the additional cup of chicken stock. Slowly braise the trimmings for 45 minutes, or until all the greens are tender (retaining the brilliant green color). Stir in the sorrel and watercress and immediately remove from the stove. Strain off half the chicken stock and reserve. Puree the asparagus greens in a blender and strain through a fine sieve. The reserved cooking liquid may be used to correct the body of the coulis.

To finish the plate:

Poach the salmon in the simmering court bouillon 10 minutes per inch of thickness. Heat up the blanched asparagus in the reserved cooking liquid from the coulis recipe. Heat up the coulis (do not boil), check for the seasoning, and add salt and white pepper to taste.

Place the salmon on a plate on the coulis and finish with 2 or 3 asparagus spears placed over the salmon.

TOMATO SAUCE

Yield: approximately 2 quarts

Ingredients:

3 cloves of garlic (peeled)
1 large Spanish onion (chopped)
½ cup carrots (chopped)
½ cup celery, (chopped)
½ cup leeks (chopped)
1 tablespoon olive oil
2 pounds plum tomatoes (chopped)
1 cup chicken stock
Basil and thyme to taste (optional)

Method:

Sauté the onion, garlic, carrots, celery, and leeks over high heat in the olive oil for approximately 10 minutes, or until tender. Add the plum tomatoes and chicken stock. Simmer for 1 hour. Strain the sauce through a fine sieve. Chill the sauce and reserve for cooking the baked spinach stuffed tomato (see following page). The remainder of the sauce may be used in other vegetable preparations, such as ratatouille.

BAKED TOMATOES STUFFED WITH SPINACH

Ingredients:

3 large tomatoes
1 tablespoon olive oil
6 cups loosely packed fresh spinach (diced)
6 cups loosely packed broccoli (diced)
1 medium onion (finely chopped)
½ cup tomato sauce (see page 179)
½ cup low-fat cottage cheese (puree in a food processor)
2 teaspoons salt
½ teaspoon white pepper
Bread crumbs

Method:

Prepare the tomatoes by removing the stems, cutting them in half, and scooping out the pulp. In a large sauté pan, sauté the onion in the olive oil over medium heat for about 5 minutes. Add the washed spinach and broccoli. Cover and steam sauté the vegetables for 8 minutes. Add the tomato sauce, cottage cheese, salt, and pepper. Cook for 5 more minutes. Generously stuff the tomato halves with spinach filling and top with the bread crumbs. Bake at 400°Fahrenheit for 10 to 15 minutes, until the bread crumbs are well browned.

STRAWBERRY MOUSSE

Ingredients:

3 cups fresh strawberries (the sweetest available)
2 tablespoons brown sugar
½ cup Neufchâtel cheese
1 cup low-fat cottage cheese
4 tablespoons "Just Whites" (mixed with water according
   to directions on the package)*
1 package plain Knox gelatin, dissolved in water

Garnish (per serving):
6 teaspoons plain low-fat yogurt
6 fresh strawberries (cut in a fan presentation)

Method:

Clean and core the strawberries, blend with the brown sugar, and let marinate for two hours. In a food processor fitted with a steel blade, puree the strawberries. Add the Neufchâtel cheese and process until the cheese is uniformly pureed with the strawberries. Then add the cottage cheese and puree again. Add the "Just Whites" and puree for uniformity. Finally add the dissolved gelatin, then pulse until thoroughly combined. Pour into 6 chilled wineglasses. Cover each with plastic wrap and refrigerate until the mousse is set. Top with the plain yogurt and strawberries when ready to serve.

Obviously, gourmet Zone-Perfect meals are not made in minutes, but they do show you how a truly gourmet meal can be created that keeps you firmly in the center of the Zone.

Note: "Just Whites" are powdered egg whites.

QUICK ZONE SNACKS

One of the biggest problems for people is finding easy-to-prepare one-block Zone snacks. Here are number of delicious choices:

LOW-FAT COTTAGE CHEESE AND FRUIT

¼ cup low-fat cottage cheese
1 block canned light fruit
1 macadamia nut or 3 almonds

TOMATO SALAD AND LOW-FAT CHEESE

3 tomatoes, diced
1 clove garlic, minced
⅓ teaspoon chopped fresh basil leaves
1 ounce low-fat cheese
⅓ teaspoon olive oil

Add balsamic vinegar to taste, then combine and mix well.

WALDORF SALAD

1 cup celery, sliced
¼ apple, diced
1 teaspoon light mayonnaise
1 pecan, crushed
1 ounce low-fat cheese

Combine and mix well.

LOW-FAT YOGURT AND NUTS

½ cup plain low-fat yogurt
1 teaspoon slivered almonds or 1 crushed macadamia nut

Sprinkle the nuts over the yogurt.

LOW-FAT COTTAGE CHEESE AND TOMATO

¼ cup low-fat cottage cheese
3 tomatoes, sliced
1 tablespoon avocado

CHEF SALAD SNACK

1½ ounces deli-style turkey or ham
1 tossed garden salad:
    2 cups shredded lettuce
    ¼ sliced tomato
    ¼ green bell pepper
    ¼ raw cucumber
    1 teaspoon olive oil and balsamic vinegar dressing:
        ⅓ teaspoon olive oil
        ⅔ teaspoon balsamic vinegar

TACO SALAD

1½ ounces ground turkey cooked with small amounts nonfat cooking spray and a small amount taco seasoning powder
1 tablespoon salsa
1 tossed green salad:
    2 cups shredded lettuce
    ¼ sliced tomato
    ¼ green bell pepper
    ¼ raw cucumber
    1 tablespoon avocado

Assemble the salad and top with cooked ground turkey and avocado.

HAM AND FRUIT

4 slices 97 percent fat-free deli ham
½ apple (or any other 1-block fruit serving)
1 macadamia nut (or any other 1-block fat)

APPLESAUCE AND LOW-FAT CHEESE

⅓ cup applesauce
1 ounce low-fat cheese
1 tablespoon avocado

BERRIES, LOW-FAT CHEESE, AND NUTS

½ cup blueberries
1 ounce low-fat cheese
1 pecan half

CHEESE AND GRAPES

1 ounce part-skim mozzarella string cheese
½ cup grapes
6 peanuts

FAT-FORTIFIED SKIM MILK

6 ounces skim milk
2 macadamia nuts or 6 almonds or 12 peanuts

COTTAGE CHEESE AND FRUIT

¼ cup low-fat cottage cheese
½ cup pineapple, diced
1 teaspoon slivered almonds

WINE AND CHEESE

4 ounces wine (or 6 ounces beer or 1 ounce distilled spirits)
1 ounce cheese

HOT DOG

1 soy hot dog
1 6-inch corn tortilla
1 teaspoon light mayonnaise or 1 tablespoon guacamole

1 PERCENT MILK

6 ounces 1 percent milk
6 peanuts

MINI PITA PIZZA

½ mini pita pocket topped with:
1 tablespoon tomato sauce
⅓ teaspoon olive oil
1 ounce part-skim mozzarella cheese

QUICK PIZZA

1 Wasa cracker topped with:
⅓ teaspoon olive oil
1 ounce low-fat cheese

Top the Wasa cracker with the olive oil and low-fat cheese and microwave on high for 30 seconds.

SPINACH SALAD

1 hard boiled egg white, sliced
1 spinach salad:
   3 cups raw spinach
   ¼ raw onion
   ¼ cup raw mushrooms
   ¼ raw tomato
   ⅓ teaspoon olive oil
   Balsamic vinegar to taste

CRABMEAT SALAD SANDWICH

1½ ounces crabmeat
1 teaspoon light mayonnaise
½ mini pita pocket cut into triangles

VEGGIES AND DIP

3 ounces firm tofu blended with ⅓ teaspoon olive oil and some
   dry onion soup mix
3 green bell peppers, sliced for dipping

CHIPS AND SALSA

½ ounce baked tortilla chips
1 tablespoon salsa
1 ounce low-fat jack cheese
1 tablespoon avocado

To make even more 1-block Zone snacks, try combinations of the following:

Proteins (choose one):
¼ cup low-fat cottage cheese
1 ounce low-fat cheese
1 ounce mozzarella cheese made with skim milk
2½ ounces ricotta cheese

Fats (choose one):
3 olives
3 hazelnuts
3 almonds
1 macadamia nut
6 peanuts
¼-inch slice of avocado

Carbohydrates (choose one):
½ apple
½ grapefruit
½ cup grapes
3 apricots
½ cup cubed honeydew melon
¾ cup cubed cantaloupe
¼ cantaloupe
¾ cup cherries
1 kiwi
½ orange
½ nectarine
1 tangerine
½ pear
1 plum
½ cup fruit cocktail
⅓ cup peaches
½ cup crushed pineapple

    1 cup strawberries
    1 cup raspberries
    ¾ cup blackberries
    ¾ cup blueberries

With meals ranging from quick Zone meals to gourmet Zone-Perfect meals to simple-to-prepare Zone snacks, you now have all the tools to enter the Zone with remarkable ease. The following chapters will give you even more tools to make your stay in the Zone a permanent one.

7

ZONING YOUR KITCHEN

Staying in the Zone becomes even easier if you take the time to Zone your kitchen so that you can quickly and easily make Zone-Perfect meals any time of the day.

Try to visualize your new Zone kitchen as your food pharmacy. Every time you open the refrigerator door you'll be pulling out a drug as powerful as any you will ever encounter. So the first thing you want to do is to temporarily remove all the potentially dangerous drugs from your kitchen that will drive you out of the Zone. Take all the pasta, rice, pancake and cookie mixes, breads, and bagels and put them in a bag. Then put the bag in the trash or in a dark corner of your basement where you aren't likely to venture in the next few weeks. Do the same for all the breadmakers and juicers you own. (It's not that juicers are bad, but they remove fiber from the fruit and make it easier to overconsume fruit in the form of juice.) Put them in the attic. That's step one, and it takes only a few minutes.

Zone-Perfect meals are primarily based on low-fat protein, fruits, and vegetables, which means grocery shopping will be a key to your success. So here's a helpful Zone hint: Buy protein, fruits, and vegetables two to three times a week. It's amazing that with all the grocery stores and automobiles available to Americans, for many of us buying food is in the same category as making a trek to Outer Mongolia. Go to the store two to three times a week to buy perishables like protein, fruits, and vegetables. Buy only what you need for the next couple of days of Zone-Perfect meals, which means you are less likely to throw out any once-fresh food bought one or two weeks earlier.

PROTEIN

Always choose low-fat sources such as chicken, turkey, very lean cuts of beef, fish, low-fat cottage cheese, or soybean-based food products. This is desirable because you are always going to add some monounsaturated fat back to your meal. Always try to have some protein already prepared in your refrigerator for easy snacking. This might include sliced turkey, cottage cheese, string cheese, tuna salad, or even a tofu dip.

CARBOHYDRATES

The carbohydrate foundation of the Zone Diet is built upon fruits and vegetables. If you think that fresh fruit and vegetables are too expensive compared to pasta, then consider using frozen fruit and vegetables. They won't taste as good, but, surprisingly, they are actually more nutritious than the fresh variety. By the time "fresh" food reaches your home, it's been on the road for a long time. It has to be picked, packed, and trucked to the distribution center. Then it is trucked again to the supermarket, where it sits until you buy it. Then you transport it to your home, where it sits again until you eat it. The longer it sits, the more nutrition (especially vitamins) is lost.

Frozen fruits and vegetables, on the other hand, lead a different life. Usually only the best food picked is quick-frozen, and this is done within hours after harvesting. The end result is that frozen fruit and vegetables will usually have a higher vitamin content by the time they get to your home than fresh fruit or vegetables.

Of course you can always purchase canned fruits and vegetables, but these are a different story nutritionally. They will be the most inexpensive, but there will be a significant drop-off in their vitamin and mineral content (and in their taste, for that matter). Yet no matter how much nutrition canned fruits and vegetables have lost, they will still have more nutrients than the freshest bagel or fanciest pasta.

FATS

Of all the basic components of the Zone Diet, fats have the longest shelf life, and cooking oils can almost be considered Zone staples because you don't have to shop continually for them to maintain their freshness.

There are three good reasons to use oils in cooking. First, the fat found in oils acts like soluble fiber to slow down the rate of entry of any carbohydrate into the bloodstream. Second, fat also sends a hormonal signal to the brain to say stop eating. Finally, fat makes food taste better and enhances the flavors of the food. Since fat has no effect on insulin, make it your ally, not your enemy, in your Zone kitchen.

Another key to Zone cooking is using oils instead of butter when you cook. Not just any type of oil, however, will do. The best oil is olive oil, because it's rich in monounsaturated fats. This type of fat has absolutely no effect on insulin, and thus will be an integral partner in your battle against obesity. Surprisingly, the best type of olive oil to cook with is not the premium extra virgin olive oil, but the considerably less expensive refined olive oil.

The terms *extra virgin* and *virgin* denote the amount of contaminants of free fatty acids (which have a bitter taste) in the olive oil. *Extra virgin* means the oil has less than 0.5 percent by weight of free fatty acids, whereas *virgin* indicates less than 1.0 percent by weight. Olive oil containing more than 2 percent of free fatty acids has to be refined, which will reduce the amount of the free fatty acid to 0 percent. That's right, a big zero. Unfortunately, refining also removes many of the components that give premium olive oil its unique flavor characteristics. Therefore, refined olive oil won't have the zesty zing with all the flavor of the more expensive brands, but as far as cooking in the Zone goes, it is the ideal one to use. Keep in mind that oils do not have an indefinite shelf life. Never keep an oil more than six months, and store it in a cool location that is not exposed to light.

FROZEN FOODS

Frozen foods should be an ideal component in a Zone kitchen because of their long shelf-life. The only problem is the taste. Freezing pulls water from the cells so that food loses its plumpness at the cellular level. As a result, food loses its texture. In addition, the formation of ice crystals in the food can damage cells and cause the loss of flavor and nutrients. This happens because water expands when it freezes and the ice crystals can act as microscopic blades. Vegetables tend to freeze better than meats, seafood, and fruit. Some vegetables, such as peas, spinach, and lima beans, usually retain a reasonable texture after thawing. On the other hand, broccoli and cauliflower don't hold up well during freezing and lose the most texture.

Here are some Zone tips on buying frozen foods. If there is any frost on the package, it means that it has been partially thawed and some of the water has escaped and has refrozen on the outside of the package. Avoid those packages. Also, take your frozen food from deep inside the freezer, since the temperature is likely to be cooler with less chance of thawing.

ZONE STAPLES

Plan to restock your kitchen with Zone staples. These are items that make Zone cooking and snacking incredibly easy. Since Zone staples have a long shelf life, measured in months, you won't have to buy these as often.

The first Zone staple to buy is oatmeal, the only grain I really recommend on the Zone Diet. It's rich in soluble fiber (known as beta-glucan) that slows down the absorption of carbohydrate, and it contains an essential fatty acid (gamma linolenic acid, or GLA) that is found in mother's breast milk. (Not surprisingly, it's also what your grandmother told you to eat for breakfast.) Oats are rich in soluble fiber, as are many fruits (like apples) and vegetables (like black beans and kidney beans). But oat manufacturers have better marketing people, so that's why the Food and Drug Administration has given them permission to label their products with the following message: "Soluble fiber from oatmeal, as part of a low saturated fat, low cholesterol diet, may reduce the risk of heart disease." Too bad the apple lobby and black bean lobby are not as powerful or as savvy as the oat lobby.

What if you don't have thirty minutes to cook oatmeal in the morning? The next best choice is old-fashioned oats, which have been steamed and rolled between large steel rollers to flatten them. These oats take about five minutes to cook, and they still retain their chewy texture.

Not all oatmeals are the same, and you pay a real hormonal price for convenience. Additional processing to raw oatmeal to make it faster to cook results in less insulin control. All oatmeals start with the whole grain known as the groat. The groat is then steamed to soften the oats. Without a doubt, these are the best oats for cooking: thick, coarse oats that take about thirty minutes to cook. These oats are also known as Scottish oats or Irish oatmeal and are the kind that I most highly recommend.

What if you don't have thirty minutes to cook oatmeal in the morning? The next best choice is old-fashioned oats, which have been steamed and rolled between large steel rollers to flatten them. These oats take about five minutes to cook, and they still retain their chewy texture.

Further processing gives you quick oats, which are simply old-fashioned oats that have been cut to allow them to cook faster (in about one minute). Unfortunately, the faster cooking time also means that the carbohydrates in the oatmeal will enter your bloodstream faster. A further significant step down in insulin control are instant oats, which are cut even finer than quick oats, and need only boiling water and a little stirring to prepare.

However, even the worst type of oatmeal (instant oats) is still superior to any other type of typical cold breakfast cereal in slowing down the rate of entry of carbohydrates into the bloodstream because of the soluble fiber content. (The typical cold breakfast cereal has only insoluble fiber, which has no effect on carbohydrate entry into the bloodstream). The slower the entry rate of carbohydrates into the blood, the less insulin you produce and the less likely it is that you'll move out of the Zone with that meal.

One protein source can be considered a Zone staple because of its very long shelf life. That source is isolated protein powder, which can be used to fortify a meal with adequate protein. Although there are many types of isolate protein powders, hormonally speaking the best is soybean isolate, as it has the least effect on insulin and the greatest effect on glucagon. Unfortunately, soybean isolates don't taste as good as other isolated protein sources such as whey, milk, or egg proteins. As with oatmeal, there will be a compromise between taste and hormonal benefits.

Another important Zone staple is nuts. Before people learned how to extract oil from olives or seeds some 5,000 years ago, they ate nuts for fat. Nuts are a great storage tank for oils. Realize that once you extract an oil from a seed or nut, it begins to go rancid very quickly. In fact, the shelf-life of a typical isolated oil under the best conditions (no exposure to air, no exposure to light, and maintained at room temperature) is only six months. Therefore the oils in nuts are much more resistant to rancidity. Your best choices are nuts rich in monounsaturated fats, like macadamia nuts and almonds. This is why slivered almonds are a great condiment to any meal. Other good choices in nuts rich in monounsaturated fats are cashews and pistachios.

Peanuts are also a readily available monounsaturated fat source, although not quite as rich in monounsaturated fat as the nuts discussed above. Although many people would like to think of peanut butter as a source of protein, in reality it's primarily a fat (although a pretty good fat). A better Zone choice would be almond butter. Using nuts or nut butters are great ways to add monounsaturated fat to Zone-Perfect meals.

The last Zone staples you definitely want in your Zone kitchen are spices. Remember, it was during the quest for cheaper access to spices that America was discovered. Spices were so highly sought because they make food taste better. The more spices you use, the greater the taste sensations. And spices have no effect on insulin. Life is good.

8

ZONE TOOLS

Now that you have Zoned your kitchen, you still need some basic Zone tools for cooking Zone-Perfect meals. Let's start with the most important—knives. A good sharp knife is your greatest Zone tool—the sharper the edge, the faster you can prepare Zone-Perfect meals.

KNIVES

By far and away the best raw material for making knives is carbon steel. Unfortunately, this material is attacked by acids (found in lemons and citrus fruits) that can stain the knife. These knives have to be wiped clean right after use to prevent staining. If you are truly a gourmet cook, carbon steel knives are your choice.

The next step down in blade sharpness are high-carbon knives. The cutting edge will not be as sharp as the edge of carbon steel knives, but these knives will not stain when exposed to acid. However, these knives are the most expensive. Companies like Henckels and Forshmer manufacture these knives.

Lower in quality and sharpness of edge is a stainless steel knife. Unlike carbon steel knives, these knives will become dull very quickly. And the duller the edge of the knife, the more effort involved in food preparation. Finally, some knives are super stainless steel. These are advertised as never needing sharpening. This is because they *can't* be sharpened. Stay away from these knives. Since a good knife should last a lifetime, make an appropriate investment for your Zone kitchen.

Once you decide which type of material you plan to choose for your knives, determine what type of knives you need. The four basic knives needed in any Zone kitchen include: a paring knife (three to four inches in length), a utility knife (six inches in length), a chef's knife (eight inches in length), and a slicing or carving knife (usually ten inches in length). The chef's knife is thicker than a slicing knife because the extra weight produces chopping power. On the other hand, the slicing knife is narrower and gives thinner slices, which is a major advantage in Zone cooking.

Now that you have the knives, buy a knife sharpener. Unless you keep the edges beveled to improve the ease of cutting (regardless of the material), you're more likely to revert to using prepared meals as it becomes more difficult and time-consuming to prepare the basic ingredients required for Zone-Perfect meals.

Keeping your knives sharp actually makes your kitchen a much safer place. Surprisingly, dull knives are more dangerous than sharp knives. First, you're likely to be more careful using a sharp knife than a dull one. Second, a sharp knife is less likely to slip since you have to apply less pressure to cut food than with a dull knife. A sharper knife also means more efficiency and quicker preparation time in the kitchen. You also minimize tearing and ripping of your protein source or vegetables, and the thinner slices mean less cooking time.

POTS AND PANS

Your next most important Zone kitchen tools are your pots and pans. Preparing the raw ingredients for Zone-Perfect meals is one thing, cooking them is another. You need the appropriate pots and pans to increase heat transfer and cook the food with the least amount of vitamin and mineral loss.

The secret of Zone cooking is not spending much time in the

kitchen, and this includes cleanup. Therefore, nonstick pans will be your greatest ally. Teflon is the first type of pan that comes to mind, but as most of you know, the Teflon coating can be easily scratched. A better choice for longevity would be Silverstone, since it lasts longer and therefore becomes less expensive in the long run. Anodized aluminum pans are another potential choice. The surface of these pans has been oxidized to prevent food from adhering, which provides them with a "nonsticky" surface.

But the reason you use metal pans is to get good, uniform heat transfer from your range to the food. When it comes to heat transfer, copper and aluminum are among the best metals. The trouble with copper is that it needs constant cleaning to prevent oxide formation, which reduces heat transfer. Stainless steel is less efficient, and glass and earthenware are the least desirable for efficient heat transfer. Stainless steel pans with a copper bottom may appear to be a good compromise, but the copper coating is actually very thin and it still needs constant cleaning and attention.

The thicker the pan, the better and more uniform the heat transfer to the food. This is why cast-iron skillets are often used by gourmet chefs. Probably the most reasonable choice in cookware is what is called a multi-ply pan. These pans have a layer of aluminum sandwiched between two layers of stainless steel. This gives you good heat transfer with a minimum of cleaning, a very important Zone kitchen feature.

In your Zone kitchen, the primary pan will be a frying or sauté pan. A sauté pan has a high vertical wall (about two and a half inches), which reduces the amount of splattering. This is different from a skillet, which has sloping walls to help slide food out of the pan. Other essential pans are various sizes of saucepans so that you can cook for one as well as for a family.

One other key item to consider for your Zone kitchen is a hanging fruit basket. Fruit will last longer if you allow air to circulate totally around the fruit. Fruits are still alive and consume oxygen even after harvesting. If oxygen is restricted, then the fruit at the cellular level switches to anaerobic (in the absence of oxygen) metabolism, causing a buildup of alcohol. This in turn causes brown spots below the skin of the fruit and brown cores within the fruit. Besides making fruit last longer, fruit baskets look great hanging from the ceiling.

9

ZONE COOKING TIPS

Now that you have Zoned your kitchen and have all your Zone tools together, here are some helpful hints for making Zone cooking an integral part of your life.

RANGES AND OVENS

As far as cooking itself goes, I believe that gas ranges and electric ovens are best for preparing Zone meals. Gas ranges will give you more control when cooking (especially in turning down the heat) than electric ranges. This is especially true if you plan to do any stir-frying. On the other hand, electric ovens provide a more constant temperature than gas ovens. A third type of oven is the convection oven, which circulates the heated air, giving even more uniform temperature control and cutting down on cooking time by about one-third. Although they are more expensive, so is your time in the kitchen.

But what about microwave ovens? Microwave cooking was invented in 1947 and represents the first major breakthrough in cooking technology in several centuries. Microwaves cook the food through excitation of the water molecules in the food. This is the most efficient heating process known and can cut your cooking time by up to 75 percent, because you are cooking the food from within as opposed to heating the outer surface and transferring the heat more slowly to the center of the food. Unfortunately, you pay a culinary price for such speed because microwave cooking can give food a dry, mushy texture. If food doesn't look good or taste good, what's the use of eating it?

Although there are drawbacks to microwave cooking as mentioned above, it has a real place in your Zone kitchen. Cook several Zone-Perfect meals on the weekend, and then freeze them. Heat them in the microwave during the week. High technology is your best friend in a Zone kitchen, especially since virtually everyone can operate a microwave oven.

COOKING PROTEIN

At the molecular level, meat is a combination of muscle fibers held together by collagen (collagen is basically like the wires that hold together a bale of cotton). As you heat protein, the collagen begins to liquefy into gelatin as the temperature of the meat increases. The secret of preparing meat perfectly is to detach the muscle fibers from one another (giving a tender taste and texture), but to retain enough of the collagen superstructure to prevent the protein from falling apart and becoming mushlike. Therefore cooking becomes the art of compromise.

This is why many people find fish so difficult to cook. It contains very little collagen compared to meat, and fish collagen turns to gelatin at a much lower temperature than the collagen in meat. Under ideal conditions, perfectly cooked fish flakes very easily (the muscle fibers are easily dissociated). However, slightly overcooking fish gives it that mushlike effect that makes even the experienced cook shudder.

The toughness of a cut of meat is determined by how much collagen it contains. Highly active muscles (like those of any good athlete) are rich in collagen. Also, the older the animal, the greater amount of collagen a piece of meat contains. Therefore the less active the animal, and the younger the animal before slaughter, the more tender the meat.

COOKING CARBOHYDRATES

The amount of protein you plan to prepare determines the amount of carbohydrate to be consumed at the same time. On the Zone Diet, this means eating primarily fruits and vegetables as your source of carbohydrates.

Fruits are easy to prepare. Just wash them, peel if necessary, and eat. A piece of fresh fruit or a fruit cocktail is a great dessert to complete a meal. Even adding a small dollop of whipped cream will have very little effect on insulin.

Vegetables, because of their low carbohydrate density, are always an excellent source of carbohydrates, but their preparation is somewhat different. Frankly, raw vegetables get tiresome after a little while. The best way to prepare vegetables is to lightly steam them. This preserves most of the vitamins and minerals while also making the vegetables more digestible since the steaming process has begun to break down the cell walls. Steaming also leaves very little mess to clean up (a very important feature in Zone cooking).

Although steaming is the best way to prepare vegetables, many people still will not eat them. I have found that the best way to ensure people (even your kids) will eat vegetables is to sauté them in olive oil. It will take some time, but it works.

Finally, keep the grains, starches, and breads to a minimum on the Zone Diet. These foods have such a dense carbohydrate content that they will cause a rapid increase in your insulin levels when eaten in excess. Although they are much cheaper than fruits and vegetables, you will actually see your food bills decrease once you start to use these high-density carbohydrates as condiments rather than as the base of your meals. Why? Because you won't be as hungry and your carbohydrate cravings will be dramatically reduced, if not eliminated, which means spending less money on snack foods.

COOKING WITH FAT

Because you are using low-fat protein sources, you can now add back the fat of your choice as a sauce or dressing, using your favorite monounsaturated fat source (like olive oil), or as condiments including olives, guacamole, macadamia nuts, or almonds. If you stir-fry tofu, for example, leave the oil in the meal when you serve it. The fat will carry the flavor of the spices and seasonings with the tofu.

ZONE COOKING

Regardless of your type of stove or oven, there are two ways to cook any food: using dry heat or using moist heat. These cooking methods have not really changed to any great extent over the centuries. Dry heat cooks the food through the air. While air is not a very good conductor of heat (this is why you can put your hand into an oven at 400 degrees Fahrenheit and not get immediately burned), you can heat it to a pretty high temperature. Obviously the earliest form of dry heating was roasting over an open fire. A more recent innovation (starting about 5,000 years ago) was baking using an oven to retain the heat. In both cases you are heating the air around the food to cook it.

Broiling is an even faster way to create heat transfer, as the surface of the heating elements can become extremely hot (3,000 degrees Fahrenheit for gas burners and 2,000 degrees Fahrenheit for electric burners), and the protein is usually only six inches away from the heating element. Not surprisingly, it is easy to overcook food when broiling, and therefore this method is used only with relatively thin and tender protein (i.e., that containing less connective tissue).

A variation of dry heating is pan-frying or sautéing. To prevent the protein from sticking to the pan, you add some oil. Since oil transfers heat very well, the addition of cooking oil can decrease the cooking time. But like broiling, less cooking time with higher heat means you run the risk of undercooking the interior of the protein while overcooking the exterior. This is why food preparation using a sharp knife to keep the food very thin and very tender is ideal for sautéing.

Stir-frying is simply sautéing with a different type of pan (with higher sloping walls and a deeper well), and is primarily used for cooking vegetables instead of protein. As in sautéing, you add a small amount of oil to prevent the food from sticking and to aid in heat transfer. In fact, the only difference between sautéing and stir-frying is the type of pan used. One reason that very little cooking oil is used in stir-frying was that until recently cooking oil was extremely expensive, whereas vegetables were very cheap. It therefore made good economic sense not to use much cooking oil. As a result, constant stirring was necessary to maintain contact of the vegetables with the thin film of oil.

Moist heating uses water instead of air to transfer the heat to the food. Although water cannot be heated as hot as air, it conducts heat much more effectively (imagine if you were to stick one hand in boiling water and the other hand in a heated oven at 400 degrees Fahrenheit) and therefore is usually used with tougher cuts of meat or very fiber-rich vegetables. Since you can't heat water beyond 212 degrees Fahrenheit, it also becomes hard (but not impossible) to overcook food (unless you boil away all the water), although you may have to cook it for a long time to break down the collagen. The less experienced a cook you are, or the cheaper the cuts of protein you use, the more I recommend that you use moist heat to cook your foods.

Boiling is the most common form of moist heat as you are surrounding the entire food with water. Unfortunately, this is also the best way to leach out all the vitamins and minerals from the food into the surrounding water. Other forms of moist cooking include simmering and stewing. Simmering simply means keeping the temperature of the liquid less than 212 degrees Fahrenheit, usually around 195 degrees Fahrenheit, whereas in stewing the meat is cut into smaller pieces and usually overcooked so the connective tissue is completely broken down, making it "fork tender."

You can also decrease the cooking time using moist heat by increasing the pressure of the water. Steaming or pressure cooking are two ways to achieve this goal, as they allow you to get to a higher temperature, and therefore cook food faster.

Braising is a compromise between stewing and sautéing because a small amount of water is added to a closed pan. This allows longer cooking without the danger of overcooking. Braising is usually used with large cuts of meat that have a lot of connective tissue, such as a rump roast.

Then there is deep-frying. This is basically boiling with oil instead of water. Now you can reach a much higher temperature (nearly 400 degrees Fahrenheit) and have great heat transfer to the food because of the intimate contact of the heated oil with the food. This is why French fries get cooked so quickly using deep-frying compared to the time it takes to bake a potato. But of course your food is now drenched in fat. While the Zone Diet recommends more fat in the diet, even I draw the line at deep-frying.

10

MAKING FOOD TASTE BETTER

The secret of French cooking has always been the sauces. Why do sauces make food taste better? It's the fat. Fat not only gives food a better mouth feel, but also carries flavors better, since most flavors are fat-soluble.

The best French sauces are essentially emulsified fat. Examples of natural emulsified fats are butter and milk. Butter is called a water-in-fat emulsion (since most of the weight is fat, with a small amount of emulsified water), whereas milk is a water-in-oil emulsion (most of the weight is water, with a small amount of emulsified fat).

The most common manmade emulsified sauce is mayonnaise. As the name suggests, mayonnaise originated in France and is often considered the poor relative of sauces, since it is used for adding fat to everything from a turkey sandwich to potato salad. More complex fat emulsions include hollandaise sauce used for vegetables like artichokes, asparagus, and broccoli, and béarnaise sauce used for meat. In fact, béarnaise sauce is actually hollandaise sauce to which tarragon leaves and tarragon vinegar have been added. Frankly, any Zone meal is going to taste better when you use these more complex fat emulsions in your meal.

Why were sauces first developed? Because food (especially protein) tasted pretty bad within a couple of days without refrigeration, and a century ago there was no refrigeration. Let a piece of beef sit out at room temperature for a couple of days and you see why sauces were so important. The best way to cover up the foul odor of rancid meat is to use a sauce of great flavor. Béarnaise sauce does a great job for steak. The fat in the sauce also adds mouth feel to your taste buds (remember that before grain was fed to livestock, most meat was very lean). Furthermore, fat holds flavor better, as most flavors are actually fat-soluble chemicals. In a fat-rich environment provided by the sauce, flavors blend together much better and retain their unique sensory impact.

Small wonder that once the French learned how to cover up rancid meat with sauces it took little time to realize that vegetables would also taste better by adding sauces to them.

When you think of sauces, like béarnaise and hollandaise, you usually envision a tub of melted butter used in the preparation of the sauce. Zone sauces are a little different. Rather than using massive amounts of butter, replace the butter with refined olive oil. Now you have the right type of monounsaturated fat that is heart healthy and has all of the flavor benefits of a classic French sauce. Combine these Zone sauces with Zone meals, and you are really cooking.

Salad dressings, like vinaigrette, are also emulsions. The emulsified oil (ideally olive oil) in the dressing will not be repulsed by the water on the surface of the lettuce in the salad, and mixes nicely.

Can sauces be used with fruits? Of course. Probably the easiest sauce for fruit is whipped cream. Whipped cream is also an emulsion. If you are going to whip the cream yourself, use the freshest possible cream, as any lactic acid (the off-flavor in milk) will tend to destroy the emulsion.

How do you make an emulsified Zone sauce in minutes? The easiest way is to buy a prepared dry hollandaise or béarnaise sauce mix at any grocery store. Take the dry mix, add one or two tablespoons of olive oil to it, and stir until the oil is fully blended in (this takes about fifteen seconds). Then add the right of amount of low-fat milk to it, and stir in a saucepan near boiling for about one to two minutes until the sauce thickens. Then pour the appropriate amount over the vegetables or the protein. Just as the French did more than two centuries ago, and are still doing today.

Although the Zoned sauces in Chapter 6 are easy to make, if you are feeling a little more adventuresome, you can try your hand at some variations of sauce recipes with the addition of other ingredients. For example, add julienne vegetables to the Zoned Espagnol Sauce to create Jardiniere Sauce. However, to make complex emulsified sauces, like hollandaise or béarnaise from scratch, you need to know a little food chemistry, and you often need a lot of luck. Once you try to make your own emulsified sauces, you realize that those packages of dry mixes are actually a pretty good idea.

If sauces are the secret of French cooking, spices and herbs can't be too far behind. Since the flavors of spices and herbs are heat-sensitive, the best time to add seasoning to a meal is just at the end of sautéing the meat or vegetables because prolonged exposure to heat will dissipate the flavors of the seasonings.

While sauces and seasonings add flavor and zest to any meal, there is one anti-spice. It's called monosodium glutamate, or MSG. The Japanese learned long ago that adding seaweed to a meal tended to increase the flavor. The active ingredient in seaweed? It's MSG. If you are really a poor cook or use inferior quality materials, MSG is your spice of choice. Whatever flavor is actually in the food will be enhanced. Unfortunately for many people, there will be a price for using this spice, because many react violently to its presence in food, probably due to MSG's potential neurotoxic effects on the central nervous system. For this reason alone, you should never use MSG, and you should steer clear of any food that may contain it.

Finally there is the ubiquitous seasoning—sugar. Sweetness is one of the four types of receptors on our taste buds. The other three are receptors for bitterness, hot, and cold. Since many plants make poisonous alkaloids as a defense, having a bitter taste receptor makes good evolutionary sense to keep you from eating such toxic plants. If a food had a sweet taste, you could be pretty sure that it was safe to eat.

Today, however, those same sweet receptors increase your likelihood of eating more food. So if you are a food manufacturer, the more sugar you put into the food, the more likely the consumer will be to eat it.

The key to staying in the Zone is to use natural sweeteners that have the least impact on insulin. This means fructose, which is about 33 percent sweeter for the same amount of carbohydrate found in table sugar. In addition, fructose enters the bloodstream very slowly as glucose because it must be converted to glucose by an enzyme (phosphofructose kinase) found in the liver. Because of the slow entry rate, it has a very limited effect on insulin secretion. This makes it the ideal Zone sweetener for any Zone kitchen. Always try to use the type of natural sweetener that has the greatest sweetness for the least amount of carbohydrate. Just for reference, although fructose is slightly sweeter than table sugar, it is twice as sweet as pure glucose (the most potent stimulator of insulin), three times as sweet as maltose, and six times as sweet as lactose (the sugar found in milk). Where do you find fructose? In every supermarket in America.

Artificial sweeteners are a different story. Saccharine is an intensely sweet-tasting compound that has been used since the 1920s to sweeten food. Although it is 700 times sweeter than sugar, it leaves a slight aftertaste that doesn't make it a very good sweetener. Unfortunately, since the 1980s saccharine has all but been replaced by a newer food additive, aspartame. This sweetener is actually two amino acids linked together to form a very small protein that interacts with the sweet taste receptors in your mouth, to generate the sensation of sweetness. Although aspartame has become ubiquitous in our society, I still have strong reservations about its massive use because of continual adverse reports to the FDA about some individuals who seem to be sensitive to it. If you can, try to avoid aspartame whenever possible.

However, there is a new sweetener that is actually an old one. It's called stevia, and it's an herbal preparation that is 300 times sweeter than sugar. Long used in Asia, it is now available in many health food stores in this country as a nutritional supplement. If you want to use an artificial sweetener, consider stevia your best bet.

KIDS IN THE ZONE

11

If you think being in the Zone is important for you, it's even more important for your kids. While adult obesity has increased by 32 percent in the last decade, the extent of childhood obesity has doubled. It's a literal epidemic, and yet no one seems to care.

I am the first to admit that kids are incredibly picky eaters. But more to your advantage, they are even worse cooks. And to top it off, they are incredibly lazy in the kitchen. You can use these realities to get your kids into the Zone. If you do, you will suddenly begin to look like the Ward and June Cleaver of your block because your kids will maintain better blood sugar levels, which means they actually begin to listen to you and their mood swings will be highly moderated. They might even start to clean up their rooms. (Maybe not!)

The easiest way to get kids in the Zone is to make Zone desserts. This isn't as hard as you think. In fact, your grandmother did it all the time using a dessert that wiggled. That dessert was natural gelatin with some fruit embedded in it. Protein from the gelatin, carbohydrate from the fruit. And the fat? Add a dab of whipped cream to it.

If you are a little more adventuresome with your desserts, try adding some protein powder to pudding. When you check the pudding package for its nutritional labeling, you come to realize that most puddings are virtually pure carbohydrate. Blend in enough protein powder to balance out the carbohydrates as you make the pudding, and presto it becomes Zone-Perfect. Again, don't be afraid to add a little whipped cream to it.

One of the biggest problems for parents is getting kids to eat protein. Well, there is one protein source that virtually every kid will eat, and it's called string cheese. String cheese is popular with kids because it looks like junk food. It also matches their cooking ability, which usually stops with opening a wrapper. String cheese may be a little high in saturated fat, but it's a very convenient and user-friendly way of getting some protein into your child. A good compromise is string cheese made from skim milk or low-fat milk. The ideal snack for many kids would be a piece of string cheese plus some carbohydrate like a cup of grapes (they don't need much preparation either).

Another trick parents can use is to make blended drinks that have the correct protein-to-carbohydrate ratio. Actually, we have one that has been around for nearly 8,000 years. It's called milk. Although it enters the bloodstream faster than solid food (and therefore will not have an optimal effect on insulin secretion), it's a great source of calcium and it's easy to make (just pour). Unfortunately, a good number of kids are lactose intolerant. This means they can't digest the carbohydrate in milk. In these cases, try soy milk, which is devoid of any lactose but still contains the correct protein-to-carbohydrate ratio.

To make milk more of a treat, think about malted milk. The malt is extra carbohydrate, so this means you have to add some extra protein powder to it to keep the drink in the Zone. But if your child is more likely to drink it, then it's worth the extra effort.

A variation on this theme is making a fruit smoothie to which you add some extra protein powder. Since a fruit smoothie requires a blender, this seemingly small task is well beyond the cooking skills of most kids. But you can make a protein-fortified fruit smoothie for your children and keep it in the refrigerator so all they have to do is pour. Now this is definitely within the range of their cooking skills.

Yogurt seems like a logical snack choice for most kids. But very few kids like natural yogurt. Food manufacturers realize this and therefore load up commercial yogurts with massive amounts of carbohydrates (either extra fruit or simply extra sugar) to make the yogurt taste better. Unfortunately, the end result for children when they eat these carbohydrate-heavy "healthy" yogurts is that they fall right out of the Zone. Frozen yogurt is even worse, because it is almost pure carbohydrate. It is simply politically correct cotton candy, especially if it's fat-free, and should be avoided unless you're having a protein chaser with it.

The food choices above are the easy part. The next step is to begin to teach your kids to eat the foods they were designed to eat—fruits and vegetables. Fruits should be great for kids since they require no cooking. But fruits can be intimidating for kids because they have to be peeled. So start your kids out with the easy fruits: grapes, apples, and pears. These don't require a lot of work on their part. But even here, if you precut the fruits for your kids, you will dramatically increase the likelihood that they will actually eat them. The same is true of oranges that have to be peeled, which for many kids is the equivalent of climbing Mount Everest. Here's the solution, but you have to do a little preparation because you will actually have to cut these fruits yourself (do you think your kids will?). Every couple of days, cut up a lot of strawberries, oranges, and melons and put them in a bowl in the refrigerator. As soon as your kids come home after school, put the bowl out and let them eat from it. What they don't eat, put back into the refrigerator. Use your kids' laziness to your advantage. Faced with the challenge of opening a package of potato chips or simply eating prepared fruit waiting for them when they come home should be a no-brainer for your child. Just make sure to have some string cheese waiting too.

The same is true with breakfast. Before they leave for school, take out the same bowl of precut fruit for them to eat. For a little variety, you can add some precut apples, pears, or other fruits that tend to oxidize quickly. Squirt a little lemon juice on the cut fruit to prevent oxidation. Nothing turns off a kid more than brown fruit. You will have to make a new fruit bowl every other day, but it sure beats buying a six-pack of potato chips or other snack goodies every week.

Regardless of the fruit you provide for your children, make sure they have easy access to a protein chaser to balance the carbohydrates in the fruit. Try your old standby of string cheese. Keep it in the wrapper, because if your kid doesn't eat it, you can always put it back into the refrigerator.

To make life easier for you, simply ask your children to make a list of what kinds of protein they will eat. It might be a very short list, but at least it's a beginning. That list might include Canadian bacon or egg-white omelettes in the morning, sliced turkey or string cheese at lunch, and chicken, fish, or very lean cuts of beef at dinner. And if your child is a vegetarian, then try soybean imitation meat products like soybean sausages for breakfast, soybean hot dogs for lunch, and soybean hamburger patties for dinner.

Of course, the greatest challenge for a parent is getting kids to eat vegetables. It was also the greatest challenge for your grandmother. One solution is to put vegetables in a soup or stew. Just make sure that you have adequate protein at the same time. Another way is to sauté vegetables in olive oil and add some spices like oregano to them. The more olive oil you use to sauté the vegetables, the more likely your kids are going to eat them. And herein lies the secret with vegetables: added fat. Sautéing vegetables in olive oil is one way. The other method is to do what the French learned to do centuries ago: add sauces. As discussed in the last chapter, the best sauces are nothing but emulsified fat that adds great taste to any vegetable or food. Even canned vegetables that have been sitting in your pantry for the past three years will taste pretty good once you put some sauces over them. And the better the quality of the sauce, the more likely that your kids will eat their vegetables without a big production at lunch or dinner.

12

ZONE SUPPLEMENTS

Macronutrients (protein, carbohydrate, and fat), not micronutrient (vitamin and mineral) supplements, are your passport to the Zone. Are supplements important for the Zone? A few are, but never let the tail wag the dog. Used properly, they can enhance the hormonal benefits of being in the Zone, but they will never get you to the Zone by themselves.

It is commonly reported that today's food supply is adulterated with pesticides, herbicides, hormones, and antibiotics. I agree. And if you are really concerned about your health, you should take every opportunity to use only organically grown fruits and vegetables, and range-fed chicken and beef. However, Americans want it both ways: safe food and cheap food. The cheapest food on the face of the earth is only made possible by using the very same substances that cause everyone justifiable concern. So while organic fruits and vegetables are available, recognize that you are going to have to pay a much higher price for them and you may have to spend much more time searching out these items. The same is true of range-fed and hormone-free chicken and beef.

I strongly recommend using unadulterated food whenever possible. Since the Zone is all about hormonal control, it doesn't take a genius to figure out that if food sources contain hormones, herbicides, or pesticides, they can have adverse hormonal effects that can push you out of the Zone. If you opt for cheaper food, then plan to pay even closer attention to the protein-to-carbohydrate ratio at every meal, which should help counteract the effects of the other substances that have been creeping into our food supply over the past fifty years.

And what about vitamins and minerals? Isn't our food poorer in these essential micronutrients than it was fifty years ago? The answer is probably yes. Why? Because fifty years ago, most of the fruits and vegetables came from your backyard or just outside town at the nearby farm. Now they come from all over the world and can be stored for months after being harvested. Vitamins are incredibly sensitive to heat, light, and storage time. Minerals are more stable, but they are very sensitive to processing and cooking technologies. The first casualties in the war for cheap food will always be the vitamin and mineral content of that food. So should you spend a good chunk of your food budget down at the local health food store? No, but you can use nutritional supplements wisely to get the most Zone bang for the buck.

ESSENTIAL SUPPLEMENTS

As I mentioned in *The Zone,* only two supplements are essential for the Zone Diet: purified fish oils and vitamin E. Both are supported by compelling research about their health benefits, and their cost is relatively inexpensive.

Let's talk about fish oil first, since your grandmother probably used this in the form of cod liver oil. Cod liver oil is rich in vitamin A and vitamin D, and two generations ago fear of a disease called rickets, caused by a deficiency of vitamin D, was still fresh in many minds. Cod liver oil was the best source for these vitamins, even though it was (and probably still is) one of the most disgusting foods known to man. Disgusting or not, its daily consumption was a given in your grandmother's day.

It turns out the real reason that cod liver oil was so beneficial was not because of the vitamins it contained, but because of a rare fatty acid called eicospentaenoic acid, or EPA. EPA turns out to be a key factor in controlling insulin levels. So even though your grandmother was forcing your parents to take cod liver oil for the wrong biochemical reason, she was doing an excellent job of controlling insulin in the process.

Just as the balance of protein to carbohydrate is critical for maintaining the Zone, so is the balance of certain types of fats called essential fats. These essential fats come in two distinct groups, Omega–6 and Omega–3. EPA is a long-chain Omega–3 fat that keeps this balance in sync. Fish are very efficient concentrators of EPA (which is made by plankton) since they are at the end of the food chain that begins with these single-celled organisms.

Although humans evolved from the sea, the need for these Omega–3 fatty acids is only now being realized. In fact, 50 percent of the fat mass of the brain is composed of these long-chain Omega–3 fats. No other organ in the body has such a concentration of Omega–3 fats. And since the greatest growth spurt for the brain occurs during the first two years of life, it's not surprising how important these Omega–3 fatty acids are for proper brain development. Human breast milk is rich in these types of fat. Just how important are these Omega–3 fats found in breast milk? One English study indicated that breast-fed children scored nearly eight points higher on IQ tests compared to children who were bottle-fed. This is why infant formula manufacturers are scrambling (at least in Europe and Japan) to try to incorporate these long-chain Omega–3 fatty acids, like EPA, into their products.

Dietary EPA is also strongly implicated in reducing heart disease, cancer, arthritis, and other chronic disease conditions in humans. Why? Because of its effect on a group of hormones called eicosanoids. Eicosanoids are described in far greater detail in *The Zone*, but simply stated, if you want to decrease the likelihood of developing chronic diseases, adequate amounts of EPA can help.

What are adequate amounts of EPA? Approximately 200 to 400 milligrams per day if you are in the Zone, much more if you aren't.

And the best source of EPA is cold-water fatty fish, like salmon, mackerel, and sardines. Eating fish is another Zone plus because fish represents a unique source of protein. Fish is the only source of protein that is low in Omega–6 essential fatty acids, and which provides relatively large amounts of long-chain Omega–3 fatty acids such as EPA. In the last eighty years, we have been consuming massive amounts of Omega–6 fatty acids while simultaneously reducing our intake of Omega–3 fatty acids. At the turn of the century, the ratio of Omega–6 to Omega–3 fatty acids was close to two to one. Now it's about twenty to one. One result of this shift in the essential fatty acid ratio is that we have created a massive eicosanoid imbalance, which is one of the key factors in the development of chronic disease. This is why eating fish has such a dramatic effect on the reduction of heart disease. First, eating fish means that you are probably eating adequate amounts of protein to help keep you in the Zone. Second, by eating fish you are consuming larger amounts of EPA. Third, you are decreasing your intake of Omega–6 fatty acids. Three very good reasons to eat fish.

However, there is a down side to eating fish. Fish are also great accumulators of chemically persistent toxins, like PCBs. These chemicals tend to be very resistant to being broken down by any species of life, and as a result accumulate at the end of the food chain. As a consequence fish oil can be rich in PCBs, even though PCB production was phased out decades ago. The solution to this dilemma is to supplement your diet with molecularly distilled fish oil. Molecular distillation is a high-tech process that removes PCBs from purified fish oil. Whether or not you like fish, I recommend molecularly distilled fish oils. They give you the EPA you need and peace of mind on the PCB issue.

The other essential supplement to the Zone Diet is vitamin E. Vitamin E was discovered in 1922 when it was found that a diet deficient in this vitamin was the cause of fetal death in pregnant rats and testicular atrophy in male rats. Vitamin E is not only a significant player in your reproductive system, but it plays a key role in virtually every aspect of human physiology. Unfortunately, it is simply impossible to obtain adequate levels of vitamin E through diet alone. As with fish oil, the data is compelling that increased supplementation with vitamin E will have a dramatic clinical effect on diseases ranging from heart disease to Alzheimer's and immune system disorders. I recommend taking a minimum of 100 International Units (IU) per day, with 400 IU as a reasonable upper limit for adults and 50 to 100 IU as a reasonable upper limit for children

The story of the manufacturing of vitamin E is a tale of our times. In the early days of vitamin E manufacturing, the raw material (which is still used), called distillate, was removed during the purification of soybean oil. This distillate was originally fed to cattle to further increase their milk production. Unfortunately, within a few months, thousands of cattle had died because it turned out this same distillate was also rich in herbicides and pesticides. Today the only way to manufacture natural vitamin E that is suitable for human consumption is to use molecular distillation to remove the fat-soluble herbicides and pesticides that contaminate the initial raw material that contains the vitamin E. To make natural vitamin E suitable for human consumption, you have to use the same high-tech process that also removes PCBs from fish oil.

SECOND TIER SUPPLEMENTS

Fish oil and vitamin E are essential supplements for the Zone Diet (and for any other diet, for that matter), but a second tier of vitamins and minerals can operate as an important and a very cheap insurance policy for anyone interested in his or her own health. This tier of supplements includes vitamin C and the mineral magnesium.

People often forget that the glory years of vitamin research were in the 1930s when several Nobel Prizes were awarded for discoveries in this field. In fact, the 1937 Nobel Prize in medicine was awarded to Albert Szent-Gyorgyi for his efforts in defining the structure of vitamin C.

Vitamin C is a water-soluble antioxidant. Most oxidation products in the body tend to be fat-soluble and therefore water-insoluble. The problem for the body is getting these water-insoluble oxidation products through the bloodstream to the liver so that they can be detoxified and excreted in the urine. This is where vitamin C comes in. Being water-soluble, it acts as the primary transporting agent to get rid of all the nasty oxidation products that are constantly being formed in your body. And if you don't have enough vitamin C, these oxidation products pile up and are stored in your fat cells, where they can cause trouble.

Fortunately vitamin C is plentiful, especially on the Zone Diet. Unlike vitamin E and purified fish oil, where supplementation is a must, fruits and vegetables tend to be rich in this vitamin. Not surprisingly, these are also key components of the Zone Diet. The best sources of vitamin C in fruits are kiwi, oranges, strawberries, and melons. Vegetable sources such as red peppers, broccoli, spinach, and mustard greens are also rich in vitamin C. Although megadoses are often touted, the best research indicates that a reasonable level for vitamin C supplementation is in the range of 500 to 1,000 milligrams per day. Because vitamin C is so inexpensive, this vitamin is a good recommendation even at these levels of supplementation.

The other supplement I highly recommended is the mineral magnesium. No mineral is as important as magnesium for the Zone Diet. It's the key mineral cofactor in the production of eicosanoids, and it is also a cofactor required for the proper function of more than 350 other enzymes. The latest research shows that adequate magnesium is critical for cardiovascular patients, which only makes it reasonable to assume that it is useful for the rest of us, especially since dietary surveys indicate that nearly 75 percent of Americans are deficient in this key mineral. Contained in chlorophyll, magnesium is found in every vegetable that is green, like spinach and peas. However, the richest naturally occurring sources of magnesium are nuts. Other sources that are relatively rich in magnesium are legumes, shrimp, crab, and, to a lesser extent, beef (cows represent the upper end of the food chain on land that begins with chlorophyll-containing grass). These foods are also the primary foods used in the Zone Diet. Perhaps not surprisingly, the foods that are poor in magnesium are starches, breads, and pasta, the new staples of the American diet. No wonder Americans are deficient in magnesium.

Store-bought magnesium supplements are difficult to take because magnesium tastes terrible, you need a lot of it, and it is poorly absorbed. So go the natural route first. Eat lots of nuts (especially those rich in monounsaturated fat like almonds and cashews), and other foods rich in magnesium. If you insist on taking store-bought supplements, the cheapest is milk of magnesia (but it tastes terrible). Capsule forms are very inexpensive because they are primarily magnesium oxide. Magnesium oxide, though it is not very soluble by itself, will become chelated (attached) to the amino acids formed during the breakdown of protein. This chelation process will facilitate the entry of magnesium into the bloodstream, but you have to take the supplement in the presence of protein for it to be effectively absorbed. Of course, you could buy magnesium that is already chelated, and take it on an empty stomach. However, you won't get a lot of magnesium in each capsule since the amino acid used to chelate the magnesium will take up much of the space and it's a lot more expensive. Regardless of the dosage form, try to take 250 milligrams of supplemental magnesium per day.

THIRD TIER SUPPLEMENTS

I think of the third tier of supplements as relatively inexpensive additional insurance policies. Their utility to an individual on the Zone Diet is limited compared to the benefits of the supplements recommended above, but third tier supplements represent peace of mind.

The first of these third tier supplements is beta carotene. Nowhere in the world of supplements is there more confusion than there is about beta carotene. Scientists always want to search for a "magic bullet" that can be put into a capsule as the essence of health. For many years beta carotene appeared to be a magic bullet. After all, many studies showed that higher blood levels of beta carotene were associated with lower risks of heart disease and cancer. The obvious conclusion was that beta carotene was the key factor in preventing both diseases, but it turned out that the scientists were looking at the trees (and a single tree, at that) instead of the forest.

No one thought for a minute that the bloodstream of healthy people contained a lot of beta carotene because they were eating a lot of fruit! After all, if you are consuming a lot of fruit, it is unlikely that you are eating a lot of high-density carbohydrates like starches and pasta. It wasn't that beta carotene had some mystical properties as researchers first thought, but simply because fruit eaters weren't consuming as many high-density carbohydrates. As a result, they were not making as much insulin as non–fruit eaters.

The mystique of beta carotene was recently diminished by two studies based on the magic bullet approach. One study focused on smokers and the other with asbestos workers; both are high-risk groups for cancer. Large research studies were undertaken to show that taking large amounts of beta carotene would prevent cancer. The trouble was that both studies indicated that the group taking beta carotene was actually developing cancer at higher rates! Had the magic bullet of beta carotene actually become a deadly dart? I don't think so, because the increase in cancer in these studies could have a simpler alternative explanation.

Beta carotene is a great antioxidant for fat-soluble free radicals. This simply means it picks up free radicals and stabilizes them before they can do some real damage. But unless removed from the body, a stabilized free radical is just trouble looking to strike. To get these free radicals out of your system, you need to have adequate levels of water-soluble antioxidants (like vitamin C) to take the fat-soluble free radical from beta carotene and transport it to the liver, where it can be metabolically emasculated and excreted. And that was the problem with the beta carotene studies: Neither added extra vitamin C to transport the beta carotene–stabilized free radicals to the liver for their final detoxification.

Is beta carotene really dangerous to your health? Of course not, and in fact it has great utility as long as the other part of the equation (vitamin C) is present at adequate levels. This is why vitamin C is *very* important as a supplement, and beta carotene is less important as a Zone supplement.

But before you go out and buy extra beta carotene supplements, try getting it from fruits like cantaloupe, and from vegetables like red peppers and spinach. And yes, carrots contain beta carotene, but unfortunately because of the structure of the carbohydrates in the carrot, they enter the bloodstream very rapidly and thus increase insulin levels, which can be worse for your health than the benefit gained by the increase in beta carotene.

Other supplements that I place into this third tier are vitamins B_3 (niacin) and B_6 (pridoxine), which are critical for the production of eicosanoids.

Lack of niacin was discovered as the cause of pellagra, which became a widespread epidemic in this country at the turn of the century when poorer populations subsisted on white flour, white rice, and sugar, products all devoid of niacin. (Not surprisingly these foods have once again become the staples of our country, but now in the form of pasta, bagels, and rice cakes). Unlike most vitamins, niacin can be produced in the body through the conversion of the amino acid tryptophan into niacin. The process is not very efficient, but it does mean that if you are eating adequate levels of protein, you will probably avert an outright deficiency of niacin. The best source of niacin remains food, and particularly those foods that are integral to the Zone Diet, including lean meat, poultry, fish, eggs, cheese, and milk. And again, while whole grains are another good source, I don't recommend them because the higher density of carbohydrates in the grains will increase insulin levels, thus outweighing any benefit of increased niacin. If you are going to supplement with niacin, then 20 milligrams per day is a good dose. With vitamin B_6 (the second of the vitamin B pair), I recommend 5 to 10 milligrams per day. These amounts of B vitamins can also be found in any decent vitamin pill.

Folic acid is another vitamin that has received research attention because of its ability to reduce both neural tube defects in children and the levels of homocysteine, a risk factor for heart disease. The name *folic acid* comes from the Latin word for leaf because that is exactly where you find this vitamin: in leafy green vegetables. Although the RDA for this vitamin is 200 micrograms per day, the most recent research (especially on heart disease), indicates that it makes sense to take at least 500 to 1,000 micrograms per day. It turns out folic acid also works with vitamins B_3 and B_6 to reduce the levels of homocysteine, another example of synergy with other vitamins (like vitamin C and beta carotene) in the body.

Also in this same tier of useful supplements are the minerals calcium, zinc, selenium, and chromium.

You are told that calcium is necessary for strong bones, since 99 percent of the calcium in your body is in your bones. But it's also needed to control muscle contraction and nerve conduction. Dairy products, including cheese, are without a doubt the best sources of calcium. Our national fat phobia has made most dairy products persona non grata, forcing many women to go out and get calcium supplements. But dairy products aren't the only sources of calcium because broccoli, cauliflower, green leafy vegetables, and calcium-precipitated tofu also provide calcium, but the calcium in these foods is not nearly as absorbable as that found in dairy products.

Another important mineral to consider is zinc. Zinc plays a critical role in the proper functioning of your immune system and in the production of eicosanoids. Not surprisingly, good sources of zinc are the building blocks of the Zone Diet, including chicken, beef, fish, oatmeal, and nuts. If you are going to supplement with zinc, 15 milligrams per day should be sufficient. As with vitamins B_3 and B_6 you will probably find this amount of zinc in a typical vitamin-mineral supplement.

Selenium is an essential component of the enzyme known as glutathione peroxidase that reduces excess free radicals. This is why selenium supplementation is useful in cancer treatment and prevention.

Food sources higher up the food chain, such as seafood and beef, tend to be rich in selenium. Nuts are also rich in selenium. I advise a dose of 200 micrograms per day; L-selenomethionine is your best store-bought choice for maximum absorption of this supplement.

Finally, the mineral chromium is part of a biochemical complex known as glucose tolerance factor. This factor makes insulin more effective in driving blood glucose into cells for use. Therefore the more chromium you have, the less insulin you need to make. This is why chromium is called a potentiator of insulin action. Unfortunately, many supplement manufacturers have touted chromium as the only thing required to lose fat or gain muscle mass. Nothing can be further from the truth. To paraphrase President Clinton's 1992 campaign slogan, "It's the insulin, stupid." Your diet will have far greater effect on insulin than any supplement. If you choose to supplement your diet with chromium, I suggest taking approximately 200 micrograms per day.

EXOTIC AND NOT SO CHEAP SUPPLEMENTS

This last group of vitamins is interesting, but only if you have money to spare. It includes lycopene, lutein, CoQ_{10}, and oligoproanthocyanidins. All tend to be antioxidants. Two of the most interesting are the carotenoids lycopene and lutein. Lycopene has been associated with a decrease in prostate cancer and is found primarily in foods with red pigments, such as tomato and watermelon. Lutein, on the other hand, is associated with a decrease in macular degeneration (which causes an ever decreasing field of vision in the eye and leads to blindness). Where do you find lutein? In green leafy vegetables and red peppers. If you want to supplement your diet with these very expensive antioxidants, try 3 to 5 milligrams per day.

Another interesting antioxidant is CoQ_{10}. This is not really a vitamin, since the body can synthesize it, but the synthesis is usually very inefficient. CoQ_{10} functions like a souped-up vitamin E and may be the last line of defense for preventing the oxidation of low-density lipoproteins (LDL), which appears to be a major factor in the development of atherosclerosis. There is also evidence of its benefit in the treatment of congestive heart failure. I recommend 5 to 10 milligrams per day.

Finally, there are the overly hyped, but nonetheless potentially useful, antioxidants known as oligoproanthocyanidins (OPC), or polyphenolics. They are the antioxidants found in grapes and are part of the bioflavanoid family that works together with vitamin C. Since bioflavanoids have some solubility in both fats and water, they make a good shuttle system to help move stabilized free radicals from fat-soluble antioxidants, such as vitamin E and beta carotene, to water-soluble antioxidants, such as vitamin C, so that the free radical can be detoxified by the liver. A good recommendation is 5 to 10 milligrams per day.

My recommendations don't mean that other vitamins and minerals aren't important to human health, because they are. But if you are following the Zone Diet, you are probably getting adequate levels of these other micronutrients.

13

WHAT THE CRITICS SAY

Are there critics of the Zone Diet? You bet there are. And for the life of me, I don't know why. After all, the Zone Diet is not new, it's basically what your grandmother told you to eat. I believe a recent article on diets in the May 1997 issue of *Vogue* magazine hits on a potential reason for the uproar: "The Zone . . . is under constant attack by registered dietitians who would be washing floors if everyone followed the Zone."

It also seems as if many "critics" of the Zone Diet have never read any of my Zone books further than the jacket cover, and consequently have little understanding of the concept of hormonal control modulated through food. Therefore, let me summarize and debunk the various criticisms that have been leveled at the Zone Diet.

1. **"It's a high-protein diet."** This is a tired refrain that attempts to link the Zone Diet to the high-protein diets of the 1970s. These high-protein diets were exactly that—excessive in protein. The advocates of these diets said, "Eat all the protein you want, just don't eat any carbohydrate." Well, you can't eat all the protein you want because your body can only metabolize a certain amount of protein at any one meal. What's that maximum per meal? About the amount of low-fat protein you can put on the palm of your hand. And before you get too excited, that amount of protein also should be no thicker

than the palm of your hand. For most males this is about four ounces of low-fat protein, and for most females it is about three ounces of low-fat protein. Any more protein at a meal will be converted to fat, since your body can't store protein. Just make sure you get that amount of protein at each of your three meals per day. The typical American male will need about 100 grams of protein per day, whereas the typical American female will need about 75 grams per day. On a typical high-protein diet, a typical male might eat 150 or more grams of protein per day, an amount of protein that is simply too much except for world-class athletes.

Furthermore, high-protein diets are very low in carbohydrate, which generates an abnormal state called ketosis. Since you are consuming more carbohydrate than protein on the Zone Diet, it is impossible ever to be in ketosis.

Frankly, there is simply no relation between the Zone Diet and the typical high-protein diet. This is shown more clearly in Figure 13–1. As you can see from this figure, on a high-protein diet you would be consuming nearly 50 percent more protein than if you were on the Zone Diet. You would also be eating 50 percent more fat, and 250 percent *less* carbohydrate.

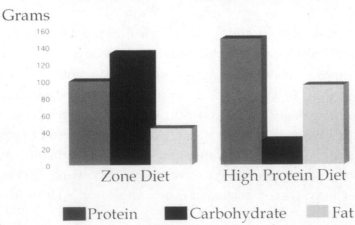

Zone Diet vs. High Protein Diet

So the Zone Diet is clearly a protein-adequate diet, not a high-protein diet, with enough carbohydrate to make it impossible to be in ketosis, but not enough carbohydrate to cause an overproduction of insulin.

2. **"A calorie is a calorie."** This is the basic mantra of most nutritionists. Weight gain and weight loss is simply a matter of calories in versus calories out. Unfortunately, this is not true for fat gain or fat loss. Gaining or losing body fat is controlled by levels of insulin. And the macronutrient makeup of a diet will have a dramatic impact on insulin levels.

As an example, if "a calorie is a calorie," shouldn't anyone on a 1,000-calorie-per-day diet lose weight? And if "a calorie is a calorie," then the composition of the calories shouldn't matter. Right? Not necessarily. One study done more than forty years ago with overweight individuals in a hospital ward setting proves this critique wrong. If "a calorie is a calorie," then weight loss would have been the same regardless of the macronutrient composition of the diet. Yet the results don't support this theory (see Figure 13–2).

In the study, when 90 percent of the 1,000 calories per day

Is A Calorie A Calorie?

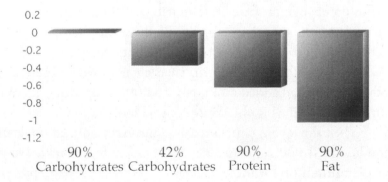

came from fat, weight loss was nearly one pound per day. This is because fat has no effect on insulin. When 90 percent of the 1,000 calories per day came from protein, weight loss was reduced to 0.6 pound per day. This is because protein has a slight stimulatory effect on insulin, but a far greater effect on the hormone glucagon that mobilizes stored carbohydrate from the liver to maintain blood sugar. When the 1,000 calories per day came from a mixed diet containing 42 percent carbohydrates (really the first published report of what has become the Zone Diet), the weight loss was reduced to about 0.4 pound per day.

Yet, when 90 percent of the 1,000 calories came from carbohydrates, the patients actually started to gain weight, even on a diet of only 1,000 calories per day! Obviously, a calorie is not a calorie when it comes to weight loss. This study is also the first published reference to what has been further refined to become the Zone Diet, because the protein-to-carbohydrate ratios were similar to those required to maintain insulin in its therapeutic zone—not too high, not too low.

The question of fat calories and weight gain was also addressed in research published in 1997 that studied the effect of adding extra fat calories to the diets of active runners. The study used athletes who ran more than thirty-five miles per week and who followed a standard diet that contained 16 percent of their calories as fat to maintain their weight at a constant level. For four weeks an extra 500 calories per day of fat were added to the runner's diet, with no change in their exercise habits. If "a calorie is a calorie," then after one month of consuming these extra fat calories, some change should have been observed in both their weight and percent of body fat. However, no such changes were observed even though they had added more than 15,000 extra fat calories to their standard diet during this four-week period.

Then the investigators increased the extra daily fat intake to an additional 1,000 calories a day for another four weeks. Now the fat consumption for these runners was equivalent to 42 percent of their calories (but their diets still maintained the same number of carbohydrate and protein calories). However, even after adding an extra 30,000 fat calories to their diet for another four weeks, there was still no change in their weight or their percent of body fat (actually they got slighter thinner).

Perhaps some nutritionist can explain to me why consuming these extra 45,000 calories of fat over an eight-week period did not increase the weight or percent of body fat in these athletes if "a calorie is a calorie"? Furthermore, the only statistically significant change was that their blood lipid profiles were significantly improved by consuming higher levels of fat, as shown in Figure 13–3. This result led the authors of the study to state that "the cardiovascular benefits of exercising by athletes may be negated by consuming a low-fat diet."

This is why the Zone Diet's focus on hormonal thinking is so different from caloric thinking.

The published medical research has shown that weight gain or weight loss is not simply a matter of fat calories in your diet. Hormonal thinking is based upon the role that excess insulin plays in making you fat and keeping you fat. And fat doesn't affect insulin.

Effects of Fat Content on Cardiovascular Risk Factors in Distance Runners

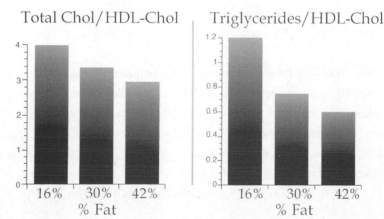

from Leddy et al *Med Sci Sports Exerc* 29: 17-25 (1997)

3. **"The Zone Diet only works because it is a low-calorie diet."**
    As research showed more than forty years ago, it is actually possible to gain weight on a low-calorie diet if it is rich in carbohydrates. The Zone Diet is a low-calorie diet that is hormonally correct. A low-calorie diet that generates high levels of insulin (i.e., a high-carbohydrate, low-fat diet) is not only hormonally incorrect, but it also represents outright deprivation. These diets are accompanied by constant hunger, fatigue, and irritability. Who wants that? The Zone Diet is very different because by keeping insulin in a tight zone, you can now access your stored energy (both fat and carbohydrate). You're not hungry on the Zone Diet because your blood sugar level is maintained by the hormone glucagon. You don't have any lack of energy because you are tapping into your stored body fat by keeping insulin levels under control. You don't have to put as many calories in your mouth if you can access your own stored body fat and stored carbohydrate. But this is only possible if you are keeping insulin in a zone.

    Obviously, at some point you can lose too much body fat. Once you reach your desired weight, you don't add any more protein since that would make your protein consumption excessive. You don't add any more carbohydrate since that would increase insulin levels. What can you add to your diet that still has calories? It's fat. You start adding more monounsaturated fat to your diet like a caloric ballast to maintain your percent of body fat, since dietary fat has no effect on insulin. In fact, the extra fat will only improve your physical performance in the Zone.

4. **"You have to be fat to be making too much insulin."** It is true that overweight individuals (especially if they have an apple shape) are producing too much insulin. But research published in 1989 in the *New England Journal of Medicine* is quite clear in pointing out that individuals with normal weight can also be hyperinsulinemic, with a resulting increase in blood pressure.

    If you are overweight, simply follow the Zone Diet to reduce insulin. If you are of normal weight and you don't want to become overweight, follow the Zone Diet. It's actually pretty simple.

5. **"There's no research to support the Zone Diet."** Actually I have already described the first published research for the prototype of the Zone Diet, which was published more than forty years ago, and another recent publication by independent investigators in 1996, which has confirmed that the Zone Diet can reduce insulin response. Furthermore, diets higher in fat and lower in carbohydrates improve the blood profiles of both Type II diabetic patients and postmenopausal women. In fact, the authors of the study on postmenopausal women stated that "it seems reasonable to question the wisdom of recommending that postmenopausal women consume low-fat, high-carbohydrate diets."

   Frankly, I am waiting for some research to appear to show that the Zone Diet doesn't work. Unfortunately, nutrition is often driven more by political agendas than by scientific facts.

6. **"The Zone Diet is too hard to follow."** If you have gotten this far in this book, then you know that statement is false. The Zone Diet is very similar to the diet your grandmother told you to eat, and all you have to do is simply balance your plate using your eyeball every time you eat.

7. **"It takes too much time to make meals on the Zone Diet."** It doesn't take long to prepare Zone-Perfect meals if you use the recipes in this book as a guide and template. And if you are really pressed for time, drive through a fast-food restaurant and create the appropriate protein-to-carbohydrate balance by throwing away any excess carbohydrate. Better yet, go to the salad bar at a local supermarket to get some fruits and vegetables, and then walk over to the deli to get some low-fat protein to balance it.

8. **"The Zone Diet is too expensive."** Yes, eating fresh fruits and vegetables instead of pasta and bagels is more expensive. But frozen fruits and vegetables are much cheaper and have more

nutrition. However, if you think the Zone Diet is expensive, then try being fat, lethargic, and prone to chronic disease as an alternative.

9. **"The Zone Diet is too radical."** Here I stand with your grandmother and the French. No one has ever accused the French of not eating well. And if the Zone Diet is radical, then everything your grandmother told you about a healthy diet is also suspect.

But the final criticism of the Zone Diet is one that I must agree with. This charge is the following:

10. **"If I am right about the Zone Diet, then virtually every nutritional expert and the U.S. government are totally wrong."** This one might be a little over the top, because in reality there is no right or wrong diet for Americans. But there are hormonally correct diets. The definition of a hormonally correct diet is one that keeps insulin in a tight zone—not too high, not too low. And whatever diet you are following, if you are keeping insulin in that Zone, then keep doing it because it's working for your biochemistry. Frankly, if you are eating Pop Tarts three times a day, and you are maintaining your insulin levels, then keep eating the Pop Tarts—although I think that's an unlikely scenario.

The Zone Diet gives you the easy-to-follow hormonal rules that allow you to achieve your goal of lifetime insulin control, and with slight modifications to your current diet it can quickly become a Zone Diet. For individuals not having success on a high-carbohydrate diet, I suggest cutting back on the high-density carbohydrates (pasta, grains, and starches), adding a little extra low-fat protein, and adding a dash of monounsaturated fat. For individuals not having success on a high-protein diet, simply cut back on the protein, add more low-density carbohydrates (fruits and vegetables) and ease off on some of the excess fat. Presto, then everyone is following the Zone Diet, and what could be simpler than that?

14

THE FUTURE OF THE ZONE

I started to develop the Zone Diet over fifteen years ago as I came to realize that conventional nutritional "wisdom" was flawed and my own future (because of my family's poor cardiovascular history) hung in the balance. Today, there is a growing body of evidence that the Zone Diet has the potential to change the very core of our health-care system as we know it. Given the direction in which our health-care system is now evolving, it seems likely that you will ultimately bear the fiscal responsibility for your own health. The days of unlimited health care are over.

Why should the Zone Diet be especially important to you now? Because in five to ten years, I believe all health care in this country will be basically controlled by the insurance companies. And what do you think will happen when they discover that the earliest indication of a potential heart attack can be measured by your insulin levels? And then what happens if your insulin levels are elevated? You can bet that eventually your insurance company is going to put you on the Zone Diet to treat your excess insulin levels, or you are going to pay much more in insurance premiums. The Zone Diet is not a fad; it is a powerful technology that can save insurance companies billions of dollars by delaying the advent of chronic diseases, such as heart disease. And money makes things happen.

What would the overall lowering of insulin levels mean for this country? One result would be a tremendous increase in the general health of the nation, despite an aging population. Another would be a giant step forward in balancing the federal budget as costs for the treatment of chronic diseases (especially Type II diabetes) would be dramatically decreased. And finally, it would mean a return to common sense in our thinking about what constitutes good nutrition.

But more importantly for you, by using the Zone Diet, you have an exceptionally powerful food pharmacy available to help you avoid chronic disease while simultaneously increasing the quality of your life. This book, and others I wrote before it, teach you how to use that pharmacy to the best advantage.

At this point, you are probably asking yourself the following questions.

1. If it is understood at the research level that elevated insulin is the primary risk factor for heart disease, why hasn't the popular press told me about this?

2. If excess carbohydrates in the diet produce excess insulin, why does the popular press tell me to eat high-carbohydrate diets?

3. If eating high-carbohydrate diets is making me fatter, why does the same popular press tell me to eat even more carbohydrates?

My answer would be "I don't know." During the last fifteen years of advocating the benefits of a high-carbohydrate diet, nothing has seemed to work despite the best efforts of the government, nutritionists, and the popular press. Americans are more confused than ever about what they should eat. I think one reason may be that when you are taught to think calorically, it is very difficult to embrace hormonal thinking. This is especially true of most of the nutritional establishment, who have made their careers by believing in caloric thinking. This is also why so many of the myths of current nutrition refuse to die.

Here are a few more myths (that you hear all the time in the popular press) that guide our current nutritional policies. They are also wrong.

1. **"A diet high in saturated fat causes heart disease."** It does if you don't eat enough fiber. But when you correct for fiber intake (increased fruit and vegetable consumption), there is no relationship between heart disease and saturated fat. This is why Spaniards, who are eating more saturated fat and fewer grains, have seen their heart disease rates drop dramatically over the past twenty years.

2. **"A diet high in very saturated fat like lard increases cholesterol levels."** Lard is considered the most potent artery-clogging food known to man (at least in the popular press). Yet when you feed the primary fatty acid found in lard (stearic acid) to humans, there is no change in total cholesterol or even LDL cholesterol levels. It turns out that some saturated fat is neutral, and some saturated fat is bad. It's a lot more complicated than you have been led to believe.

3. **"Pasta is the ideal health food."** What you are not told is that excess consumption of pasta is associated with increased cancer risk. In fact, a growing body of evidence links increased insulin levels to cancer, just as increased insulin levels are linked to heart disease.

4. **"Complex carbohydrates decrease diabetes."** Not really true. It very much depends on the glycemic index of the carbohydrate. The slower the rate of entry of a carbohydrate into the bloodstream, the less likely you are to develop diabetes. And the carbohydrates with the lowest glycemic index are the ones recommended on the Zone Diet. But the Zone Diet is not about the glycemic index of carbohydrates, but the insulin index of a meal.

5. **"A high-carbohydrate diet rich in pasta, starch, and breads and low in protein prevents hypertension."** In reality, a higher pro-

tein intake coupled with an increase in fruits and vegetables reduces hypertension.

Despite the mass of myths, I still believe the hormonal truth will win in the end. And the implications of the Zone are not confined just to our country or to the developed world. Contrary to popular opinion, the three major causes of death in the undeveloped world are heart disease, cancer, and stroke—just as they are in the United States. Therefore, if the Zone Diet can reduce the chronic diseases that threaten to cripple our health-care system, the same benefits can be expected for health care worldwide.

This doesn't mean eating more animal protein, just more low-fat protein. And the cheapest, most renewable source of protein is soybeans. Simply grow more soybeans, isolate the protein, and fortify the most basic meals (usually consisting of bread, rice, or corn) with adequate levels of a vegetarian source of protein (i.e., isolated soy protein), and overnight world health will be improved.

But before you can change the world, you have to change yourself. All it takes is the commitment to understand hormonal thinking, and the ability to make Zone-Perfect meals. Now that you have read this book, you can begin the process.

Welcome to the Zone.

APPENDIX A

TECHNICAL SUPPORT

The Zone is constantly evolving based on new research, new insights, and continuing feedback from users of the Zone technology. As a consequence the best method of being updated on the Zone is through our web site at http://www.eicotech.com. This web site should be used as an on-line Zone news center with updated medical research news, new Zone recipes, helpful Zone hints, and a community message board devoted to the Zone Diet.

If you don't have a computer, give us a call at 1-800-233-3426 for more information.

ZONE FOOD BLOCKS

The concept of Zone food blocks gives a straightforward method for constructing Zone meals. Listed below are the sizes of various blocks of protein, carbohydrate, and fat each consisting of one block. The protein blocks are for uncooked portions. Although favorable carbohydrates are usually low-glycemic carbohydrates, there are exceptions (like ice cream and potato chips) which are also high in fat.

I have rounded off the blocks to convenient sizes for easy memory. This list is by no means meant to be exhaustive. If you have a favorite food not listed, simply refer to Corinne Netzer's "Complete Book of Food Counts" (Dell Books) to expand the list.

Use of the Zone Food Blocks is easy. The first step is to determine the amount of protein you plan to eat at a meal. For most males this will be four blocks of protein, and for most females it will be three blocks. Then go to the protein section of Zone Food Block guide and pick out the amount of protein you need for that number of blocks. This could be a single protein source or a combination of protein sources.

Then go to the carbohydrate section of the Zone Food Block guide, and pick out an equal number of carbohydrate blocks. Likewise, this could be a single carbohydrate source or a combination of several.

Finally go the fat section of the Zone Food Block guide and

choose an equal number of fat blocks. The final ratio of protein, carbohydrate, and fat blocks in your meal should always be in 1:1:1. Since you should also be consuming two one-block snacks (one in the late afternoon and the other before retiring), this means the average male should consume about fourteen blocks per day and the average female eleven blocks per day. I personally recommend that every adult consume at least eleven blocks per day.

PROTEIN BLOCKS (APPROXIMATELY 7 GRAMS PROTEIN PER BLOCK)

Meat and Poultry

Best Choices

Chicken breast, skinless	1 ounce
Chicken breast, deli-style	1½ ounces
Turkey breast, skinless	1 ounce
Turkey breast, deli-style	1½ ounces
Veal	1 ounce

Fair Choices

Beef, lean cuts	1 ounce
Beef, ground (10 to 15 percent fat)	1½ ounces
Canadian bacon, lean	1 ounce
Chicken, dark meat, skinless	1 ounce
Duck	1½ ounces
Corned beef, lean	1 ounce
Ham, lean	1 ounce
Ham, deli-style	1½ ounces
Lamb, lean	1 ounce
Pork, lean	1 ounce
Pork chop	1 ounce
Turkey, dark meat, skinless	1 ounce
Turkey bacon	3½ slices

Poor Choices

Bacon	3½ slices
Beef, fatty cuts	1 ounce
Beef, ground (less than 15 percent fat)	1½ ounces
Hot dog (pork or beef)	1 link
Hot dog (turkey or chicken)	1 link
Kielbasa	2 ounces
Liver, beef	1 ounce
Liver, chicken	1 ounce
Pepperoni	1 ounce
Salami	1 ounce

Fish and Seafood

Bass	1½ ounces
Bluefish	1½ ounces
Calamari	1½ ounces
Catfish	1½ ounces
Cod	1½ ounces
Clams	1½ ounces
Crabmeat	1½ ounces
Haddock	1½ ounces
Halibut	1½ ounces
Lobster	1½ ounces
Mackerel*	1½ ounces
Salmon*	1½ ounces
Sardine*	1 ounce
Scallops	1½ ounces
Snapper	1½ ounces
Swordfish	1½ ounces
Shrimp	1½ ounces
Trout	1½ ounces
Tuna (steak)	1½ ounces
Tuna, canned in water	1 ounce

(Source: *Rich in EPA)

Eggs

Best Choices

Egg whites	2
Egg substitute	¼ cup

Poor Choice

Whole egg	1

Protein-Rich Dairy

Best Choice

Cottage cheese, low fat	¼ cup

Fair Choices

Cheese, reduced fat	1 ounce
Mozzarella cheese, skim	1 ounce
Ricotta cheese, skim	2 ounces

Poor Choice

Hard cheeses	1 ounce

Vegetarian

Tofu, soft	3 ounces
Protein powder	⅓ ounce
Soy burgers	½ patty
Soy hot dog	1 link
Soy sausages	2 links

MIXED PROTEIN/CARBOHYDRATE (Contains one block of protein and one block of carbohydrate)

Milk, low fat (1 percent)	1 cup
Yogurt, plain	½ cup
Tempeh	1½ ounce

CARBOHYDRATE BLOCKS (APPROXIMATELY 9 GRAMS OF CARBOHYDRATE PER BLOCK)

Favorable Carbohydrates

Cooked Vegetables

Artichoke	1 medium
Asparagus	1 cup (12 spears)
Beans, green or wax	1 cup
Beans, black	¼ cup
Bok choy	3 cups
Broccoli	1¼ cups
Brussels sprouts	1½ cups
Cabbage	1⅓ cups
Cauliflower	2 cups
Chickpeas	¼ cup
Collard greens	2 cups
Eggplant	1½ cups
Kale	1 cup
Kidney beans	¼ cup
Leeks	1 cup
Lentils	¼ cup
Mushrooms (boiled)	1 cup
Onions (boiled)	½ cup
Okra, sliced	1 cup
Sauerkraut	1 cup
Spinach	1 cup
Swiss chard	1 cup
Turnip, mashed	1 cup
Turnip greens	1½ cups
Yellow squash	1 cup
Zucchini	1½ cups

Raw Vegetables

Alfalfa sprouts	11 cups
Bean sprouts	3 cups
Bamboo shoots	2 cups
Cabbage, shredded	3 cups
Cauliflower	2 cups
Celery, sliced	2½ cups
Cucumber	1
Cucumber, sliced	4 cups
Endive, chopped	7½ cups
Escarole, chopped	7½ cups
Green peppers	3
Green pepper, chopped	2¼ cups
Humus	¼ cup
Lettuce, iceberg	1½ heads
Lettuce, romaine, chopped	6 cups
Mushrooms, chopped	3 cups
Onion, chopped	1 cup
Radishes, sliced	2 cups
Salsa	½ cup
Snow peas	1 cup
Spinach	6 cups
Spinach salad (2 cups raw spinach, ¼ raw onion, ¼ raw mushrooms, and ¼ raw tomato)	1
Tomato	2
Tomato, chopped	1¼ cups
Tossed salad (2 cups shredded lettuce, ¼ raw green pepper, ¼ raw cucumber, and ¼ raw tomato)	1
Water chestnuts	⅓ cup

Fruits (fresh, frozen, or canned light)

Apple	½
Applesauce	¼ cup
Apricots	3
Blackberries	¾ cup
Blueberries	¾ cup
Cantaloupe	¼ melon
Cantaloupe, cubed	¾ cup
Cherries	¾
Fruit cocktail	½ cup
Grapes	½ cup
Grapefruit	½
Honeydew melon, cubed	½ cup
Kiwi	1
Lemon	1
Lime	1
Nectarine	½
Orange	½
Orange, Mandarin canned	⅓ cup
Peach	1
Peaches, canned	½ cup
Pear	½
Pineapple, cubed	½ cup
Plum	1
Raspberries	1 cup
Strawberries	1 cup
Tangerine	1
Watermelon	¾ cup

Grains

Oatmeal (slow cooking)**	⅓ cup (cooked)
Oatmeal (slow cooking)**	½ ounce dry

(Source: **contains GLA)

Unfavorable Carbohydrates (use in moderation)

Cooked Vegetables

Acorn squash	½ cup
Baked beans	⅛ cup
Beets, sliced	½ cup
Butternut squash	⅓ cup
Carrots, sliced	½ cup
Corn	¼ cup
French fries	5
Lima beans	¼ cup
Parsnip	⅓
Peas	⅓ cup
Pinto beans	⅓ cup
Potato, baked	⅓ cup
Potato, boiled	⅓ cup
Potato, mashed	⅕ cup
Refined beans	¼ cup
Sweet potato, baked	⅓
Sweet potato, mashed	⅕ cup

Fruits

Banana	⅓
Cranberries	¼ cup
Cranberry sauce	3 teaspoons
Dates	2 pieces
Fig	1 piece
Guava	½ cup
Kumquat	3
Mango, sliced	⅓ cup
Papaya, cubed	½ cup
Prunes (dried)	2
Raisins	1 tablespoon

Fruit Juices

Apple juice	⅓ cup
Apple cider	⅓ cup
Cranberry juice	¼ cup
Fruit punch	¼ cup
Grape juice	½ cup
Grapefruit juice	⅓ cup
Lemon juice	⅓ cup
Lemonade	⅓ cup
Orange juice	⅓ cup
Pineapple juice	¼ cup
Tomato juice	¾ cup
V–8 juice	¾ cup

Grains and Breads

Bagel (small)	¼
Barley	½ tablespoon
Biscuit	¼
Bread crumbs	½ ounce
Bread, whole grain	½ slice
Bread, white	½ slice
Breadstick	1
Buckwheat, dry	½ ounce
Bulgur wheat, dry	½ ounce
Carrot	1
Carrot, shredded	1 cup
Cereal, dry	½ ounce
Cornbread	1 square
Cornstarch	4 teaspoons
Couscous	½ ounce
Croissant, plain	¼
Crouton	½ ounce
Donut, plain	¼

English muffin	¼
Granola	½ ounce
Grits, cooked	⅓ cup
Melba toast	½ ounce
Millet	½ ounce
Muffin, blueberry	¼
Noodles, egg (cooked)	¼ cup
Pancake (four-inch)	½
Pasta, cooked	¼ cup
Pita bread	¼ pocket
Pita bread, mini	½ pocket
Popcorn, popped	2 cups
Rice, brown (cooked)	⅕ cup
Rice, white (cooked)	⅕ cup
Rice cake	1
Roll, bulky	¼
Roll, dinner	½ small
Roll, hamburger	¼
Taco shell	1
Tortilla, corn (six-inch)	1
Tortilla, flour (eight-inch)	½
Waffle	½

Others

Barbecue sauce	2 tablespoons
Candy bar	¼
Catsup	2 tablespoons
Cocktail sauce	2 tablespoons
Crackers (saltine)	4
Cracker (Graham)	1
Honey	½ tablespoon
Jam or jelly	2 teaspoons
Ice cream, regular	¼ cup
Ice cream, premium	⅙ cup

Molasses	2 teaspoons
Plum sauce	1½ tablespoons
Potato chips	½ ounce
Pretzels	½ ounce
Relish, pickle	4 teaspoons
Sugar, brown	1½ teaspoons
Sugar, granulated	2 teaspoons
Sugar, confectionery	1 tablespoon
Syrup, maple	2 teaspoons
Syrup, pancake	2 teaspoons
Teriyaki sauce	½ ounce
Tortilla chips	½ ounce

FAT (APPROXIMATELY 1½ GRAMS PER BLOCK)

Best Choices (rich in monounsaturated fat)

Almond butter	⅓ teaspoon
Almonds (slivered)	1 teaspoon
Almonds	3 teaspoons
Avocado	1 tablespoon
Canola oil	⅓ teaspoon
Guacamole	1 tablespoon
Macadamia nut	1
Olive oil and vinegar dressing	1 teaspoon
Olive oil	⅓ teaspoon
Peanut oil	⅓ teaspoon
Olives	3
Peanut butter, natural	½ teaspoon
Peanuts	6
Tahini	½ tablespoon

Fair Choices (low in saturated fat)

Mayonnaise, regular	⅓ teaspoon
Mayonnaise, light	1 teaspoon

Sesame oil	½ teaspoon
Soybean oil	⅓ teaspoon

Poor Choices (rich in saturated fat)

Bacon bits (imitation)	2 teaspoons
Butter	⅓ teaspoon
Cream	½ tablespoon
Cream cheese	1 teaspoon
Cream cheese, light	2 teaspoons
Lard	⅓ teaspoon
Sour cream	½ tablespoon
Sour cream, light	1 tablespoon
Vegetable shortening	⅓ teaspoon

APPENDIX C

REFERENCES

Acherio A, Rimm EB, Giovannucci EL, Spegelman D, Stampfer M, and Willett WC. "Dietary fat and risk of coronary heart disease in men." Brit Med J 313: 84–90 (1996)

Addison RF, Zinck ME, Ackman RG, and Sipos JC. "Behavior of DDT, polychlorinated biphenyls and dieldrin at various stages of refining of marine oils for edible use." J Am Oil Chemists Soc 55: 391–394 (1978)

Addison RF. "Removal of organochlorine pesticides and polychlorinated biphenyls from marine oils during refining and hydrogenation for edible use." J Am Oil Chemists Soc 53: 192–194 (1974)

Allred JB. "Too much of a good thing? An over-emphasis on eating low-fat food may be contributing to the alarming increase in overweight amount US adults." J Am Dietetic Assoc 95: 417–418 (1995)

Alpha-tocopherol Beta-carotene Cancer Prevention Study Group. "The effect of Vitamin E and Beta-carotene on the incidence of lung cancer and other cancers in male smokers." New Engl J Med 334:1150–1155 (1996)

American Heart Association. Heart and Stroke Facts: 1996 Statistical Supplement.

251

Appel LJ, Moore TJ, Obarzanek E, Vollmer WM, Svetkey LP, Sacks FM, Bray GA, Vogt TM, Cutler JA, Windauser MM, Lin P-H, and Karanja N. "A clinical trial of the effects of dietary patterns on blood pressure." N Engl J Med 336: 1117–1124 (1997)

Arsenian MA. "Magnesium and cardiovascular disease." Progress in Cardiovascular Diseases 35: 271–310 (1993)

Baggio E, Gandini R, Plancher AC, Passeri M, and Camosino G. "Italian multicenter study on the safety and efficacy of coenzyme Q10 as adjunctive therapy in heart failure." Molec Aspects Med 15: S287-S294 (1994)

Blayrock, RL. Excitotoxins. The taste that kills. Health Press. Santa Fe, NM (1994)

Campbell LV, Marmot PE, Dyer JA, Borkman M, and Storlien LH. "The high-monounsaturated fat diet as a practical alternative for non-insulin dependent diabetes mellitus." Diabetes Care 17: 177–182 (1994)

Crawford MA and Marsh DE. The Driving Force: Food, Evolution, and the Future. Harper and Row. London. (1989)

Crawford MA, Cunnane SC, and Harbige LS. "A new theory of evolution." In Essential Fatty Acids and Eicosanoids. Sinclair A and Gibson R eds. American Oil Chemists' Society Press. Champaign, IL (1993)

Daviglus ML, Stamler J, Orencia AJ, Dyer AR, Liu K, Greenland P, Walsh MK, Morris D, and Shekelle RB. "Fish consumption and the 30-year risk of fatal myocardial infarction." N Engl J Med 336: 1046–1053 (1997)

Denke MA and Grundy SM. "Effects of fats high in stearic acid on lipid and lipoprotein concentrations in men. Am J Clin Nutr 54: 1036–1040 (1991)

Despres JP, Lamarche B, Mauriege P, Cantin B, Dagenais GR, Moorjani S, and Lupen PJ. "Hyperinsulinemia as an independent risk factor for ischemic heart disease." N Engl J Med 334: 952–957 (1996)

Eades MA. The Doctor's Complete Guide to Vitamins and Minerals. Dell. New York, NY (1994)

Flatt JP. "Use and storage of carbohydrate and fat." Am J Clin Nutr 61: 952S–959S (1995)

Franceschi S, Favero A, Decarli D, Negri E, La Vecchia C, Ferraroni M, Russo A, Salvini S, Amadori D, Conti E, Montella M, and Giacosa A. "Intake of Macronutrients and risk of breast cancer." Lancet 347: 1351–1356 (1996)

Garg A, Bonanome A, Grundy SM, Zhang ZJ, and Unger RH. "Comparison of a high-carbohydrate diet with a high-monoun-saturated fat diet in patients with non-insulin-dependent diabetes mellitus." N Engl J Med 319: 829–834 (1988)

Garg A, Grundy SM, and Koffler M. "Effect of high carbohydrate intake on hyperglycemia, islet function, and plasma lipoproteins in NIDDM." Diabetes Care 15: 1572–1580 (1992)

Garg A, Bantle JP, Henry RR, Coulston AM, Griven KA, Raatz SK, Brinkley L, Chen I, Grundy SM, Huet BA, and Reaven GM. "Effects of varying carbohydrate content of diet in patients with non-insulin-dependent diabetes mellitus." JAMA 271: 1421–1428 (1994)

Giovannucci E, Ascherio A, Rimm EB, Stampfer MJ, Colditz GA, and Willett WC. "Intake of carotenoids and retinol in relation to risk of prostate cancer." J Nat Canc Inst 87: 1767–1776 (1995)

Golay KL, Allaz AF, Morel Y, de Tonnac N, Tankova S, and Reaven G. "Similar weight loss with low- or high-carbohydrate diets." Am J Clin Nutr 63: 174–178 (1996)

Heini AF and Weinsier RL. "Divergent trends in obesity and fat intake patterns: an American paradox." Am J Med 102: 259–264 (1997)

Hillman H. Kitchen Science. Houghton Mifflin. Boston. (1989)

Hollenbeck C and Reaven GM. "Variations in insulin-stimulated glucose uptake in healthy individuals with normal glucose tolerance." J Clin Endocrin Metab 64: 1169–1173 (1987)

Jeppesen J, Schaaf P, Jones C, Zhou M-Y, Chen YD, and Reaven, GM. "Effects of low-fat, high-carbohydrate diets on risk factors for ischemic heart disease in postmenopausal women." Am J Clin Nutr 65: 1027–1033 (1997)

Katan MB, Grundy SM, and Willett WC. "Beyond low-fat diets." N Eng J Med 337: 563–567 (1997)

Kekwick A and Pawan GLS. "Calorie intake in relation to body-weight changes in the obese." Lancet ii: 155–161 (1956)

Kekwick A and Pawan GLS. "Metabolic study in human obesity with isocaloric diets high in fat, protein, or carbohydrate." Metabolism 6: 447–460 (1957)

Kern PA, Ong JM, Soffan B, and Carty J. "The effects of weight loss on the activity and expression of adipose-tisue lipoprotein lipase in very obese individuals." Metab 32: 52–56 (1990)

Laws A, King AC, Haskell WL, and Reaven GM. "Relationship of fasting plasma insulin concentration to high-density lipoprotein cholesterol and triglyceride concentrations in men." Arteriosclerosis and Thrombosis 11: 1636–1642 (1991)

Lieb CW. "The effect of an exclusive, long-continued meat diet." JAMA 87: 25–26 (1926)

Lieb CW. The effects on human beings of a twelve-month exclusive meat diet." JAMA 93: 20–22 (1929)

Lands WEM. Fish and human health. Academic Press. Orlando, FL. (1986)

Lanting CI, Fidler V, Huisman M, Touwen BCL, and Boersma ER. "Neurological differences between 9-year-old children fed breast-milk or formula-milk as babies." Lancet 344: 1319–1322 (1994)

Leddy J, Horvath P, Rowland J, and Pendergast D. "Effect of a high or low fat diet on cardiovascular risk factors in male and female runners." Med Sci Sports Exerc 29: 17–25 (1997)

Lucas A, Morley R, Cole TJ, Lister G, and Leeson-Payne C. "Breast milk and subsequent intelligence quotient in children born preterm." Lancet 339: 261–264 (1992)

McCully KS. "Vascular pathology of homosystemia: implications for the pathogenesis of arteriosclerosis." Am J Pathol 56: 111–1128 (1969)

McGee H. On Food and Cooking. MacMillan Publishing. New York. (1984)

Mohr A, Bowry VW, and Stocker R. "Dietary supplementation with coenzyme Q10 results in increased levels of ubiquninol–10 within circulating lipoproteins and increased resistance of human low-density lipoproteins to the initiation of lipid peroxidation." Biochem Biphys Acta 1126: 247–254 (1992)

Murray CJL and Lopez AD. "Mortality by cause for eight regions of the world." Lancet 349: 1269–1276 (1997)

Norman AW and Litwack G. Hormones. Academic Press. San Diego, CA (1987)

Nygard O, Nordehaug, JE, Refsum H, Ueland PM, Farstad M, and Vollset SE. "Plasma homocysteine levels and mortality in patients with coronary heart disease." New Engl J Med 337: 230–236 (1997)

Omenn GS, Goodman GE, Thornquist MD, Balmes J, Cullen MR, Glass A, Keogh JP, Meyskens, FL, Valanis R, Williams JH, Barnhart S, and Hammar S. "Effects of a combination of beta-carotene and vitamin A on lung cancer and cardiovascular disease." New Engl J Med 334: 1150–1155 (1996)

Parillo M, Rivellese AA, Ciardullo AV, Capaldo B, Giacco A, Genovese S, and Riccardi G. "A high-monounsaturated fat/low-carbohydrate diet improves peripheral insulin sensitivity in non-insulin-dependent diabetic patients." Metabol 41: 1373–1378 (1993)

Rasmussen OW, Thomsen C, Hansen KW, Vesterlund M, Winther E, and Hermansen K. "Effects on blood pressure, glucose, and lipid levels of a high-monounsaturated fat diet compared with a high-carbohydrate diet in non-insulin dependent diabetic subjects." Diabetes Care 16: 1565–1571 (1993)

Rimm EB. Stampfer MJ, Ascherio A, Giovannucci E, Colditz GA, and Willett WC. "Vitamin E consumption and risk of coronary heart disease in men." New Engl J Med 328: 1450–1456 (1993)

Roberts HJ. Aspartame. Is it Safe? Charles Press. Philadelphia, PA (1990)

Robertson RP, Gavarenski DJ, Porte D, and Bierman EL. "Inhibition of in vivo insulin secretion by prostaglandin E1." J Clin Invest 54: 310–315 (1974)

Robertson RP. "Prostaglandins, glucose homeostasis and diabetes mellitus." Ann Rev Med 43: 1–12 (1983)

Salmeron J, Manson JE, Stampfer MJ, Colditz GA, Wing AL, and Willett WC. "Dietary fiber, glycemic load, and risk of non-insulin-dependent diabetes mellitus in women." JAMA 277: 472–477 (1997)

Sears B. The Zone. Regan Books, NY (1995)

Sears B. Mastering the Zone. Regan Books, NY (1997)

Selhub J, Jacques PF, Bostom AG, D'Agostino RB, Wilson PWF, Belanger AJ, O'Leary DH, Wolf PA, Schaefer EJ, and Rosenberg IH. "Association between plasma homocysteine concentrations and extracranial carotid-artery stenosis." N Engl J Med 332: 286–291 (1995)

Serra-Majem L, Ribas L, Tresserras R, and Salleras L. "How could changes in diet explain changes in coronary heart disease mortality in Spain? The Spanish paradox." Amer J Clin Nutr 61: 1351S–1395S (1995)

Seddon JM, Ajani VA, Sperduto RD, Hiller R, Blair M, Burton TC, Farber MD, Gragoudas ES, Haller J, and Miller DT. "Dietary carotenoids, vitamins A, C, and E and age-related macular degeneration." JAMA 272: 1413–1420 (1994)

Stampfer MJ, Hennekens CH, Manson JE, Colditz GA, Rosner B, and Willett WC. "Vitamin E consumption and the risk of coronary disease in women." New Engl J Med 328: 1444–1449 (1993)

Stampfer MJ and Malinow MR. "Can lowering homocysteine levels reduce cardiovascular risk?" N Engl J Med 332:328–329 (1995)

Steinberg D, Parthasarathy S, Carew TE, Khoo JC, and Witztum JL. "Beyond cholesterol-modification of low-density lipoproteins that increase its atherogenicity." New Engl J Med 320: 915–924 (1989)

Wolever TMS, Jenkins DJA, Jenkins AL, and Josse RG. "The glycemic index: methodology and clinical implications." Am J Clin Nutr 54: 846–854 (1991)

Zavaroni I, Bonora E, Pagliara M, Dall'aglio E, Luchetti L, Buonanno G, Bonati PA, Bergonzani M, Gnudi L, Passeri M, and Reaven G. "Risk factors for coronary artery disease in healthy persons with hyperinsulinemia and normal glucose tolerance." N Engl J Med 320: 702–706 (1989)

INDEX